Revalidation: A journey for nurses and midwives

Revalidation: A journey for nurses and midwives

Marianne Fairley-Murdoch and
Paula Ingram

 Open University Press

Open University Press
McGraw-Hill Education
8th Floor
338 Euston Road
London
NW1 3BH

email: enquiries@openup.co.uk
world wide web: www.mheducation.co.uk

and Two Penn Plaza, New York, NY 10121-2289, USA

First published 2017

A catalogue record of this book is available from the British Library

ISBN-13: 978-0-33-526142-0
ISBN-10: 0-33-526142-6
eISBN: 978-0-33-526143-7

Library of Congress Cataloging-in-Publication Data
CIP data applied for

Typeset by Transforma Pvt. Ltd., Chennai, India
Printed and bound by CPI Group (UK) Ltd, Croydon, CR0 4YY

Praise for this book

"Revalidation: A journey for nurses and midwives *is a brilliant resource for today's nursing and midwifery workforce. This book provides practical guidance and solutions for practitioners and confirmers using case studies from a variety of different environments, and encourages CPD, lifelong learning, and reflection. The 'time outs' in each section are very thought provoking and allow the practitioner to relate the principles of revalidation and 'The Code' to their daily nursing practice. This book also facilitates practitioners to become more self-aware of their learning style and approach to learning, thereby assisting them to gain a deeper understanding of the way they learn best. A real practical resource which nurses and midwives from a variety of settings will find valuable."*

Lorraine Malcolm, registered nurse and teacher, UK

"Revalidation has become a bit of a scary word in the profession with nurses and midwives often feeling stressed by the perceived demands. This book helps to debunk some of the myths around the process. The authors have laid out in clear fashion the process and the requirements for each of the steps needed to demonstrate suitability to remain on the register.*

The book is structured in an accessible way and is designed to really assist registrants through the process. I particularly like the frequent activities built in as the reader progresses through the chapters."

Professor Ian Murray, Head of School of Nursing and Midwifery, Robert Gordon University, UK

"This book, which I found an informative and easy read, will dispel many of the concerns around revalidation and will be welcomed by those who view the process as a minefield to be navigated.*

When we are anxious, we tend to absorb little information, but this book with its sequential chapters and the ability it gives the reader, as the authors suggest, to dip in and out if they wish will be a useful and timely addition to the information currently provided for nurses and midwives about revalidation. Each chapter has a relevant introduction and concise summary and includes learning objectives, time out sessions, a quiz or two, pause for thought boxes and case studies. Ending the chapters with key points is I feel beneficial to its readers. The section on adult learning is a relevant addition because information about revalidation doesn't always focus on this subject in any great depth and, in my experience, there are a lot of nurses and midwives who have never given thought to their learning styles which has disadvantaged them in terms of their practice and professional development.

Not everyone, depending on where they work, has been or kept themselves informed about the revalidation process. There are many reasons for this including it not being a priority for them in the short to medium term, a feeling it will 'go away', or that others will tell them what to do, with some being unfortunate enough to work in organizations that do not see that they have a role in supporting their staff to revalidate but expect them to 'just get on with it'. This well referenced book de-mystifies the process and is, I believe, a useful resource for nurses and midwives and the organisations they work in. For those familiar with the revalidation process, the book will reinforce what they know, but there will also be, I'm sure, some learning within its pages for them too."

Annette Lobo, Consultant Midwife and
Supervisor of Midwives, NHS Fife, UK

"I found this book very easy to read, it contains an understandable explanation of everything required and gives a logical and easy to follow set of prompts. It shows clearly how to incorporate revalidation into our practice and make it as stress-free as possible!"

Myrna Melville, Registered General Nurse, UK

Contents

Acknowledgments

Thanks to Morag Gardner (Associate Director of Nursing – Acute Services) and Kathryn Brechin (Head of Nursing – Quality) for their support and encouragement to write this book and for involving me in the preparation for revalidation at both a strategic and operational level. Thanks also to NHS Fife for providing some of the examples which have been adapted and utilized throughout this book.

Introduction

Revalidation

Revalidation is the standard that all nurses and midwives in the UK and overseas need to meet from 1 April 2016 to maintain their registration with the Nursing & Midwifery Council (NMC); it replaces the previous Post-Registration Education and Practice (PREP) requirements. Every NMC registrant will need to revalidate every three years and register for an NMC Online account to confirm when they are due to revalidate. If they have a disability which makes accessing NMC Online problematic, or require extenuating circumstances to be taken into account, then the NMC have specific advice relating to this; check the NMC website for the most up-to-date information (https://www.nmc.org.uk). Remember that the online NMC revalidation declaration is due on the first of the month that you are due to re-register – e.g., if your registration is due by 31 October your revalidation due date is 1 October.

Who is this book for?

This book is for all UK and overseas NMC registrants who are required to revalidate in order to continue practising. This is applicable to all nurses and midwives practising in a variety of settings – for example the NHS, private sector, universities or social care organizations. It may be of particular benefit to those who have not engaged in any aspect of revalidation until now, or those who are newly qualified. This book may also benefit registrants who are not in a traditional nursing or midwifery role – for example, management or policy. If you are an employer of nurses and midwives, several of the sections in this book will be useful in helping you to support registrants to revalidate.

This book covers all aspects of revalidation and each chapter can be read in order, or you can 'dip in and out' of sections you are most interested in. Each chapter offers opportunities for further reflection in the *Pause for Thought* and *Time Out* activities, which can not only be used as evidence to meet the revalidation requirements but may also enhance your personal and professional development. These activities are designed to encourage reflection on your learning needs, develop your self-awareness, and explore key aspects of good practice when working with colleagues and patients, or service users. This book can help expand your knowledge of how you learn, undertake reflection, and ask for feedback. While the revalidation process is important, the key is to develop your practice so that revalidation becomes part of everyday practice and you live by the NMC Code (NMC 2015a).

The Code NMC (2015a)

The Code was revised in March 2015 to reflect the changing needs of nurses, midwives and the public (NMC 2015a), and this is further explored in Chapter 2. The NMC stated that:

> For the many committed and expert practitioners on our register, this Code should be seen as a way of reinforcing their professionalism. Through revalidation, you will provide fuller, richer evidence of your continued ability to practise safely and effectively when you renew your registration. The Code will be central in the revalidation process as a focus for professional reflection. This will give the Code significance in your professional life, and raise its status and importance for employers.
>
> (NMC 2015a: 3)

Although the NMC are clear that revalidation is an individual registrant's responsibility, employers will also have a vested interest in ensuring the continued registration of the nursing workforce. Therefore, it is worth checking via your employer to see if there are any educational workshops or preparatory events that you can attend when preparing to re-register and meet the revalidation requirements, which are displayed in Figure 1.1. This book will cover the main components

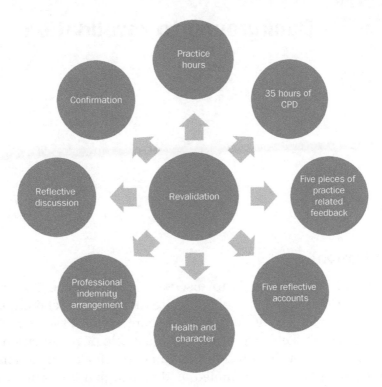

Figure 1.1 Revalidation overview

and related aspects, but you must regularly check the NMC website for the most up-to-date information as this is likely to evolve over time.

Revalidation is an individual journey and this book is designed to support and complement the revalidation process with ideas and suggestions to assist nurses and midwives. It should be remembered that the Nursing & Midwifery Council (NMC) is the 'single source of truth' and will provide all the necessary templates and forms. They will always have the most up-to-date guidance, and their guidance should be your primary reference point.

The purpose of this book is to explore the key requirements for revalidation and develop your understanding of some of these areas – for example, understanding your learning style to help you engage in continuous learning in practice, engaging in reflection, and seeking feedback. This book can be used for revalidation purposes, but hopefully also inspire further personal and professional growth resulting in improved practice.

2 Background to revalidation

Introduction

The aim of this chapter is to discuss the role of the Nursing & Midwifery Council and the role of professionalism in relation to the NMC revalidation requirements. This chapter will serve as a clear, easy-to-navigate summary of the main aspects of revalidation and the implications of this on the individual and for organizations. It incorporates practical tips aimed at demystifying the process and making it more linear for practical application. The chapter also highlights the requirements of revalidation as being the responsibility of each individual registrant.

This book must be read in conjunction with the NMC Code (NMC 2015a) and other up-to-date revalidation guidance available on the NMC website, including completed templates and case studies.

Learning objectives

By the end of this chapter you will be able to:

- Explain the role of the NMC.
- Explore perceptions of professionalism.
- Describe how the revised Code (NMC 2015a) supports revalidation.
- Discuss the NMC revalidation standards.
- Reflect and prepare for revalidation.

Professionalism

Registrants have a respected position in society and their work gives them privileged access to the public, some of whom may be very vulnerable. Being able to call yourself a professional is the advantage that comes with registration with a professional body. The role of a registrant comes with an obligation to act in accordance with certain legal, ethical and moral standards which are expected 24 hours a day, 7 days a week, 365 days of the year. The public expect certain standards of professionalism and behaviour from a registrant, and this standard is higher than that of someone who is not registered. This is because registrants are in a position of trust and responsibility and their behaviour at all times must justify the trust the public places in the profession.

Time Out

Consider how the public perceive the nursing and midwifery profession.

What impact has negative or positive press had on the public perception of the profession?

Reflect on what attributes they would expect you to possess as a professional?

How closely do you meet these attributes?

The way the public perceive nurses and midwives has an impact on the reputation of the profession, both positively and negatively. Negative media coverage, such as fitness-to-practise hearings being reported in the public domain can undermine public confidence in the profession.

Attributes of a professional

A profession should collectively demonstrate a number of elements through the acts or actions of its individual members. According to the Chief Nurse for Scotland (The Scottish Government 2012), professionalism incorporates the range of attributes and characteristics shown in Figure 2.1.

To practise safely, nurses and midwives must be competent in what they do. They must establish and maintain effective relationships

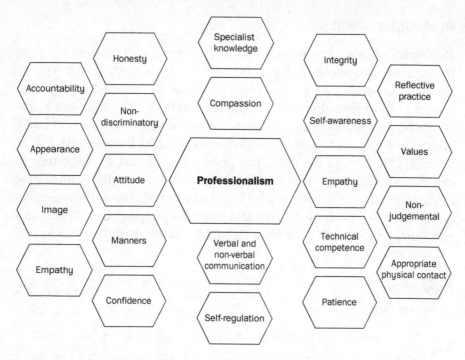

Figure 2.1 Professional attributes

with patients and colleagues. This also means that, as a registered nurse or midwife, you will act autonomously and are ultimately responsible for your actions.

Professional regulation

There are around 686,000 registered nurses and midwives in England, Wales, Scotland and Northern Ireland; they make up the largest number of registered healthcare professionals in the UK (NMC 2015b). The Nursing & Midwifery Council (NMC) has been the regulatory body for nursing and midwifery since 1 April 2002. It superseded the United Kingdom Central Council for Nursing, Midwifery and Health Visiting (UKCC) which was established in 1983. The NMC has a statutory regulatory role to protect the public, which includes upholding and sustaining confidence in the profession. The legal basis for the NMC's powers comes from the Nursing and Midwifery Order (2001), and these powers can only be amended or revoked by Parliament. This legal framework sets out the role and remit of the NMC; they are the only body who can prevent a nurse or midwife from practising.

Regulators need to be independent of government, the professionals themselves, employers, educators, and all the other interest groups involved in healthcare. The focus of regulation is as much about sustaining, improving and assuring the professional standards of the overwhelming majority of health professionals as it is about identifying and addressing poor practice or bad behaviour. However, the role of a regulator is overwhelmingly to uphold proper professional standards which is necessary for the reputation of the profession.

The NMC have a broad role in protecting the public and set professional standards to uphold the trust and confidence that patients, the public and the profession have in nursing and midwifery.

The NMC

1   Set standards of education, training, conduct and performance so that nurses and midwives can deliver high-quality healthcare throughout their careers.
2   Make sure that nurses and midwives keep their skills and knowledge up to date and uphold our professional standards.
3   Have clear and transparent processes to investigate nurses and midwives who fall short of NMC standards.
4   Maintain a register of nurses and midwives allowed to practise in the UK.

(NMC 2015b)

The standards of care expected by members of the public are greater than they used to be, with the public generally better informed. There is greater accountability to be the best professional you can possibly be.

The Code: Professional standard

The Code: Professional Standards of Practice and Behaviour for Nurses and Midwives (NMC 2015a) represents the professional standards that all nurses and midwives must uphold. 'The Code', as it is known, is a document not just for nurses and midwives but also for members of the public, including patients and relatives. It was revised in March 2015 to reflect the changing needs of nurses, midwives and the public, and has a greater emphasis on public protection. Every registrant is expected to know and uphold the fundamental tenets of the profession outlined within the Code (NMC 2015a). Working by these principles on a daily basis will ensure you meet the standards expected of your practice.

The Code (NMC 2015a) has four sections, sometimes referred to as the '4Ps':

1   Prioritise People
2   Practise Effectively
3   Preserve Safety
4   Promote Professionalism and Trust.

When the Code (NMC 2015a) was revised, a number of new areas were added. These include:

- Fundamentals of care.
- Conscientious objection.
- End of life care.
- Duty of candour.
- Social media.
- Medicines management and prescribing.

Time Out

Other useful NMC professional guidance or standards you may want to reflect on include:

- Raising concerns: guidance for nurses and midwives (NMC 2015c).
- The professional duty of candour (GMC and NMC 2015).
- Social networking guidance (NMC 2015d).
- Standards for medicine administration (NMC 2008a).

Read one of these standards. How do you meet this within your practice? Reflect on one aspect you wish to improve upon and create an action plan to achieve this.

Remember: you can use this for your revalidation evidence as this could be counted as individual learning for continuing professional development (CPD) purposes.

'Code' or 'No Code' quiz

This quiz is a fun way of testing how well you know the revised Code (NMC 2015a). The answers and an explanation are given below.

For each statement, decide whether this is in the Code or not; either 'Code' or 'No Code'.

1   You must share all necessary information with patients and other healthcare professionals and agencies when requested.
2   You must check people's understanding from time to time to keep misunderstanding or mistakes to a minimum.
3   You must be supportive of colleagues who are encountering health or performance problems.
4   Make sure you do not express your personal beliefs (including political, religious or moral beliefs) to people in your care.
5   You must provide honest, accurate and constructive feedback to colleagues when asked.
6   You must always refuse to treat a patient or service user if it is against your beliefs.
7   You must refrain from providing or engaging in care provision for a complaint until the complaint is resolved.
8   You must deal with differences of professional opinion with colleagues by discussion and informed debate, respecting their views and opinions and behaving in a professional way at all times.

Answers

1   NO CODE: but this links to the Code Section 5.5: 'Share with people, their families and their carers, as far as the law allows, the information they want or need to know about their health, care and ongoing treatment sensitively and in a way they can understand.' (NMC 2015a: 6).
2   CODE Section 7.4: 'Check people's understanding from time to time to keep misunderstanding or mistakes to a minimum.' (NMC 2015a: 8).

3   CODE Section 8.7: 'Be supportive of colleagues who are encountering health or performance problems. However, this support must never compromise or be at the expense of patient or public safety.' (NMC 2015a: 8).

4   NO CODE: but this links to the Code Section 20.7: 'Make sure you do not express your personal beliefs (including political, religious or moral beliefs) to people in an inappropriate way.' (NMC 2015a: 15).

5   CODE Section 9.1: 'Provide honest, accurate and constructive feedback to colleagues.' (NMC 2015a: 8).

6   NO CODE: but see the Code Section 4.4: 'Tell colleagues, your manager and the person receiving care if you have a conscientious objection to a particular procedure and arrange for a suitably qualified colleague to take over responsibility for that person's care.' (Note that conscientious objection can only be made in limited circumstances – e.g. termination of pregnancy, Human Fertilisation Act) (NMC 2015a: 6).

7   NO CODE: See Section 24.1, which is the exact opposite: 'Never allow someone's complaint to affect the care that is provided to them.' (NMC 2015a: 18).

8   CODE Section 9.3: 'Deal with differences of professional opinion with colleagues by discussion and informed debate, respecting their views and opinions and behaving in a professional way at all times.' (NMC 2015a: 9).

Time Out

Consider your answers to this quiz. How well do you know what is contained within the Code? You may wish to share your observations with colleagues.

Remember to record any activities as CPD which may be counted towards your revalidation evidence (see also Chapter 4).

Historical renewal of registration

The Post-Registration Education and Practice (PREP) handbook was first published in 2001 and then updated over the years until the last update in 2011 (NMC 2011). The PREP standards set out what was legally required by the NMC in order to renew your registration. There were two main standards: the PREP practice hours standard, where at least 450 hours of practice had to be completed; and the PREP continuing professional development (CPD) standard, where at least 35 hours of continuing professional development had to be completed. The reliance was on the registrant to comply with these standards, although there was no way of verifying that this had been completed or what evidence had been obtained. The NMC audited a percentage of these portfolios; however, this was small in proportion to the number of registered nurses.

The UK government identified a need for all registered healthcare professionals to demonstrate their ongoing fitness for practice and produced the White Paper: Trust, Assurance and Safety – The Regulation of Health Professionals in the 21st Century (UK Government 2007). This paper aimed to ensure professional regulation would be reformed and was fit for purpose following the recommendations of several inquiries, including the Fifth Report into the Shipman Inquiry (Crown 2004). There was an expectation from the regulators and the public that all registrants keep themselves up to date; however, this was not felt to be sufficient to protect the public. This was because when a registrant qualified their name was placed on the relevant part of the register and remained there, unless a definite reason came to light for their removal.

Trust, Assurance and Safety – The Regulation of Health Professionals in the 21st Century (UK Government 2007)

In this White Paper the key areas to be addressed were:

1   Assuring independence: governance and accountability as professional regulators. In order to exercise their functions effectively and command the confidence of patients, the public and the professions, they need to be seen to be independent and impartial in their actions.

2   Revalidation: ensuring continuous fitness for practice. New proposals were made to ensure that all the statutorily regulated

health professions have in place arrangements for the revalidation of their professional registration through which they can periodically demonstrate their continued fitness to practise.

3   Tackling concerns to ensure greater fairness and openness in the handling of cases in which a health professional's fitness to practise is called into question.

4   Education and the role of regulatory bodies, to ensure they continue to be responsible for the educational standards of the professionals they regulate.

What is revalidation?

Revalidation is the process that allows you to maintain your registration. The Code sets out the professional requirement for all registrants that they must revalidate. Section 22 of the Code (2015a: 17) states:

> Fulfil all registration requirements. To achieve this, you must:
>
> 22.1 meet any reasonable requests so we can oversee the registration process
>
> 22.2 keep to our prescribed hours of practice and carry out continuing professional development activities, and
>
> 22.3 keep your knowledge and skills up to date, taking part in appropriate and regular learning and professional development activities that aim to maintain and develop your competence and improve your performance.

Revalidation seeks to ensure the Code (NMC 2015a) is a live document used in and on practice. Working by these principles on a daily basis will help you revalidate. It is important you are familiar with the Code, which should form the foundation of your practice.

Revalidation was introduced on 1 April 2016 and is a system of ensuring all nurses and midwives meet a range of requirements to demonstrate that they are keeping themselves up to date and practising safely and effectively (NMC 2015e). This has superseded the NMC PREP Standards (NMC 2008b) which involved completing a notification of practice form declaring you had met the required standards with no third-party verification. The NMC revalidation requirements have built on these PREP standards to ensure a more robust system and process, whereby every registrant will need to demonstrate their ongoing fitness for practice. Revalidation is not a one-off event; it is a continual process which will take place throughout your career, as part of your three-yearly renewal of registration.

Revalidation has been introduced because it promotes greater professionalism among nurses and midwives and also improves the quality of care that patients receive by encouraging reflection on practice against the revised Code (NMC 2015e). Other healthcare professionals, such as doctors, pharmacists and allied health professionals, already have their own systems of revalidation. Each professional regulatory body has approached this in a slightly different way, but with the same goal of enhanced public protection. There has been a shift in the roles and responsibilities of registrants over time, with blurring of boundaries and new and emerging professional roles. Revalidation has been introduced to enhance the professional status of nurses and midwives (NMC 2015e).

Pause for Thought

You will not be able to remain registered with the NMC unless you comply with the NMC revalidation standards.

This is your individual responsibility.

Fitness for practice

Revalidation is the way registrants will 'live' the Code (NMC 2015a); the purpose is to ensure ongoing fitness for practice. Fitness *for* practice is not the same as fitness *to* practise, which is about a registrant's suitability to remain on the register without restriction. Revalidation will not replace existing fitness to practise processes or procedures and it should not be used as a method of removing a registrant from the register. Revalidation is about celebrating good practice and adherence with professional standards; it should not be used as a tool for exposing or trying to address poor practice. It is anticipated, however, that revalidation will help many registrants to identify areas of their practice that require additional learning or improvement.

Fitness to practise

Any concerns about a registrant's fitness to practise should be raised immediately; it is not appropriate to wait until a registrant is due to revalidate to raise these concerns. Revalidation does not replace existing employer capability processes or procedures, and is not a way of highlighting deficiencies in practice. These should be managed locally using existing policies and procedures. Equally, a registrant subject to capability or fitness to practise proceedings should not be prevented from revalidating, provided they have not been removed from the register and can meet the revalidation requirements (NMC 2015e).

Pause for Thought

If a nurse or midwife is being investigated by their employer or by the NMC this will not prevent them from revalidating, providing they have met the standards for revalidation.

(NMC 2015e)

Benefits of revalidation (individuals, organizations and patient care)

The benefit of revalidation is the ability to demonstrate that you are fit to practise as a registered nurse or midwife.

Time Out

Consider the different ways revalidation will benefit individuals, the organization and the public.

While undertaking the Time Out activity you may have considered the following:

Individual benefits

- Greater ownership.
- Pride.
- Increased awareness of professional responsibilities.
- Deeper learning.
- Opportunity to participate in a reflective discussion about your practice.
- Raise awareness of the Code.

Organizational benefits

- Skilled, knowledgeable registrants.
- Encourage a culture of sharing, reflection and development.
- Improve public confidence in the profession.

Public benefits

- Better quality of care.
- Improved patient safety.
- Improved trust and confidence in the profession.
- Reassurance that registrants are keeping themselves professionally up to date.

NMC revalidation model

The NMC revalidation model was provisionally agreed by the NMC Council in December 2014 following a period of extensive consultation. This was then piloted across the UK from January to June 2015, and an evaluation of this was undertaken. The NMC Council then met on 8 October 2015 and agreed the revalidation model detailed in Figure 2.2.

450 practice hours (covered in more detail in this chapter)

Practice hours relate to where you use your nursing and/or midwifery skills and can include clinical and non-clinical roles. This is often referred to as your 'scope of practice'.

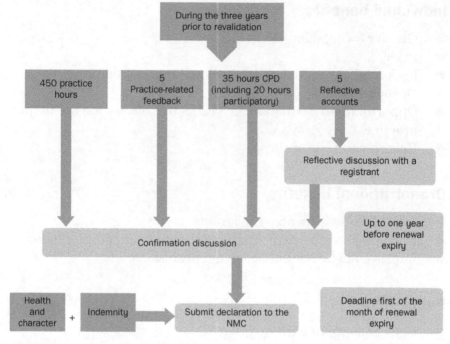

Figure 2.2 Revalidation model

Five pieces of practice-related feedback (see Chapter 5)

This is five pieces of feedback you or your team have received in relation to your practice, which can be formal or informal.

35 hours of continuing professional development, including 20 hours of participatory learning (see Chapter 4)

Continuing professional development is about the learning activities you undertake to keep up to date with your practice; these have to contain a minimum number of 20 participatory learning hours.

Five reflective accounts (see Chapter 6)

This is five written reflective accounts where you will reflect on your CPD and/or practice-related feedback, and/or an event or experience in your practice, and how this relates to the Code (NMC 2015a).

Reflective discussion (see Chapter 7)

This is where you will discuss your five reflective accounts with another registrant.

Confirmation discussion (see Chapter 9)

This is where your evidence for revalidation and renewal of your registration will be confirmed by a third party.

NMC register

The NMC register only has three parts to it: Registered Nurse (RN), Registered Midwife (RM) and Specialist Community Public Health Nurses (SCPHN).

The registered nurse part of the register is split into two subparts. Subpart 1: nurses have undertaken three-year direct entry training or one-year post-registration training leading to qualification in the fields of learning disabilities, mental health, adult or children's nursing.

Subpart 2: nurses have undertaken two-year training leading to qualification as a second-level nurse in learning disabilities, mental health, adult, general or fever nursing. These nurses used to be known as Enrolled Nurses, but are now entitled to call themselves Registered Nurses provided they can practise in this role competently. Registration as a second-level registered nurse ceased to be available for nurses training from 1992 onwards in the UK; however, some EU/EEA programmes still equate to this part of the register (NMC 2016a).

The SCPHN Part 3 of the register covers any registrant practising as a family health nurse, school nurse, health visitor, occupational health nurse or specialist community public health nurse.

The NMC have provided a template to record your practice hours; for the most up-to-date template, please visit the NMC website. The hours stated in Table 2.1 are unchanged from PREP requirements and are the minimum hours you must undertake to renew your registration and meet the NMC's revalidation requirements. These practice hours do not have to be undertaken in the

Table 2.1 Revalidation practice hours

Registered Nurse Part 1	450 hours
Registered Midwife Part 2	450 hours
Registered Nurse and Specialist Community Public Health Nurses (SCPHN) Part 3	450 hours
Registered Midwife and Specialist Community Public Health Nurses (SCPHN) Part 3	450 hours
Dual registration: e.g. Registered Nurse and Registered Midwife	900 hours (450 hours nursing practice and 450 hours midwifery practice).

(NMC 2015e)

UK to count towards the 450 hours required for revalidation (NMC 2015e).

Clinical roles

Clinical practice has a very broad meaning and can refer to many different areas in which registrants may work. Clinical roles are not necessarily providing direct patient care, but are usually based within a clinical environment. Examples may include working as a staff nurse, senior charge nurse, nurse within the military defence services, clinical midwifery manager, telehealth nurse practitioner, community midwife or public health nurse.

Although you may consider your role to be clinical, not all of your time will be spent delivering direct patient care. You may be spending some of your time completing audits, delivering education, developing policy or undertaking research.

Non-clinical roles

You may be employed in a non-clinical role such as education, policy or management where you are not delivering direct patient care. If you work in a non-clinical role you can still undertake practice hours; if your role requires professional registration with the NMC then your working hours will usually count towards your practice hours.

You do not have to have an employment contract which explicitly expresses the need for nursing and/or midwifery registration. However, you must be able to demonstrate that you are using your nursing and/or midwifery knowledge and skills within your role (NMC 2015e).

Examples of non-clinical roles are midwifery lecturer, nurse educator, practice educator, nurse researcher, clinical trainer, nurse manager and policy developer.

You must consider whether you use your knowledge, skills and abilities as a registrant within your role. If you work in a different field of practice to your original registration you must ensure you work within the limits of your competence (NMC 2015a).

When considering your role, and whether it meets the NMC requirements, it is worth dividing it into areas or Pillars of Practice (See Table 2.2).

The four Pillars of Practice are:

1   Clinical Practice.
2   Leadership and Management.
3   Facilitation of Learning.
4   Evidence, Research and Development.

(The Scottish Government 2008)

These pillars reflect the information required under scope of practice on the relevant NMC practice hours template provided on the NMC website. You may not have to give details of every practice hour if you work full-time, but you must be able to describe the dates you worked, your scope of practice and work setting, across your working week or, if you do regular hours, your working year.

Your CPD must relate to your practice hours; for example, if you are working in a management role your confirmer would expect to see evidence relating to this within your revalidation evidence. If you have changed roles during your three-year renewal period then you may have a mixture of practice hours which should also be reflected in your CPD, practice-related feedback and reflective accounts.

Table 2.2 Pillars of Practice and example activities

Pillar of Practice	Example activities
Clinical Practice	Decision-making and problem-solving skills.
	Communication skills.
	Assessing and managing risk.
Leadership and Management	Negotiating and influencing.
	Workforce planning.
	Managing teams/shifts.
	Team development.
	Change management.
Facilitation of Learning	Work-based learning.
	Mentorship.
	Teaching (to colleagues, service users, patients and students).
	Coaching.
	Developing the learning environment.
Evidence, Research and Development	Audit.
	Research.
	Service improvement work.
	Publications.
	Conference presentations.

(The Scottish Government 2008)

Case study 1

Monika Gray is a senior nurse. She recognizes that not all of her work is about delivering direct patient care, and spends about 30 per cent of time doing managerial tasks within the ward. She can count all of her practice hours as she is using her knowledge and skills as a nurse, and this role is within her scope of practice.

If Monika or her confirmer were unsure they could contact the NMC for advice.

Case study 2

Jo Lee works as a researcher in a university, and she recognizes that she also uses her nursing knowledge and skills when interviewing participants and reviewing case notes. She spends 20 per cent of her time doing this, so Jo uses this to calculate her practice hours: 37.5 hour week, 7.5 hours using her skills x 60 weeks = 450 hours.

If Jo or her confirmer were unsure they could contact the NMC for advice.

Dual registration

It is important that you maintain your competency in both parts of the register. This only applies if you are a registered nurse and a registered midwife. This will be demonstrated through the evidence of practice hours for each part for which you are registered. You will only have one renewal date for both registrations and one renewal of registration when you will revalidate. Select the role you work the most hours with to choose your reflective discussion partner and/or confirmer (see Chapters 7, 8 and 9). You only need to complete one revalidation process (NMC 2015e).

Case study 3

Eliza O'Brien is a team leader in community. She is an adult nurse, a public health nurse and a practice teacher, and wonders if she will need to provide evidence for revalidation, including practice hours for all three of her roles.

Eliza should only need to provide evidence of one set of practice hours – e.g. 450 covering SCPHN/Nursing; however, it would be expected that her CPD documentation, practice-related feedback and reflective accounts would cover her three roles.

If Eliza or her confirmer was unsure about this they could contact the NMC for advice.

Case study 4

Vikram Ghatak is a child nurse on part 1 of the register, but he now works in adult cardiology and is unsure if he can maintain his registration requirements.

Vikram must ensure his CPD reflects his practice. Some registrants will have a mixture of evidence: for example, he started work in a children's ward for two years and then moved into adult cardiology for one year, so his CPD, practice-related feedback and reflective accounts may be varied. Vikram should make sure his revalidation evidence covers both areas he has practised in over his three-year cycle. He is not required by the NMC, through revalidation, to demonstrate his children's nursing practice is up to date, but would be required to demonstrate this if he wanted to return to work in that field. So it would be in his best interests to keep his CPD in this area up to date.

If Vikram or his confirmer were unsure they could contact the NMC for advice.

Renewal of registration

You are required to renew your registration every three years, and this is different to paying your annual fee. An annual retention fee is required to maintain your registration, and your registration will not be renewed until your payment is made. Remember to keep the NMC up to date with your contact details, including your email address and any payment details (NMC 2015e).

The difference between revalidation and renewal is that your renewal date is when you are due to renew your registration as part of your three-yearly cycle. Revalidation is the process whereby these requirements are achieved. You will still pay your annual fee every year. Registrants pay an annual retention fee to be retained on this register and have to apply for renewal of their registration every three years (NMC 2015e).

NMC Online

The only way you can renew your registration is by using NMC Online. This is the system you need to enrol on to be able to revalidate. It is an online portal and you will have to register for a login and password. Keep these details safe as you will be required to use these to log in and complete your renewal of registration and revalidation information. The portal will allow you to check when your annual fee is due and when you are due to revalidate. The NMC will use the email address registered with NMC Online to communicate with you, so make sure you check your junk mail on a regular basis, particularly if you are using a personal email account. There is no requirement to use the email address related to your employment (if you have one); it is entirely up to you which email address you decide to use, but whichever one you do register, make sure you access it on a regular basis.

The NMC revalidation requirements: what this means for you

Each of the NMC revalidation requirements are presented in Figure 2.3 as a quick reference guide. Table 2.3 contains details of the requirements and a description of how you may want to meet each of the requirements.

Remember: these have to be completed over the three years prior to the renewal of your registration.

There is also a checklist to work through at the end of this chapter giving you advice for success in your revalidation.

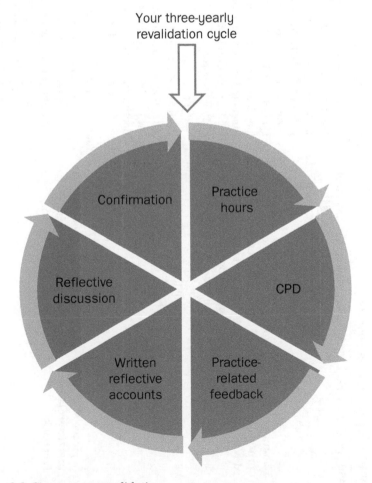

Figure 2.3 Six steps to revalidation

Table 2.3 Meeting the NMC revalidation requirements

NMC revalidation requirements	A guide to meeting these requirements
450 practice hours You must practise a minimum of 450 hours or 900 hours if revalidating as a nurse and midwife.	You will be asked to declare that you have worked the minimum hours required as a registrant. Your practice hours will relate to your own specific scope of practice and are not limited to direct patient care. You may be asked to provide written evidence of these hours. Your confirmer will want to see this.
35 hours continuing professional development You must undertake 35 hours of continuing professional development (CPD) relevant to your scope of practice. Of these hours, a minimum of 20 must be through participatory learning.	CPD must be relevant to your practice; at least 20 hours must be 'participatory', which means you have to have interacted with others to learn either, physically or virtually, e.g. clinical training, conference or webinar. You should record: • The CPD method. • A brief description of the topic and how it relates to your practice. • Dates the CPD activity was undertaken. • The number of hours and participatory hours. • Identification of the part of the Code most relevant to the CPD. • Evidence of the CPD activity. Your confirmer will want to see this.
Five pieces of practice-related feedback You must obtain at least five pieces of practice-related feedback.	You may not always need to seek feedback. It is likely that you will already receive a range of feedback: for example, from colleagues, students, patients, appraisal or through reviewing complaints and serious event reviews. You will have to be able to explain the feedback you have received to your confirmer, so the NMC recommend that you keep a note of the content of the feedback and how you used it to improve your practice.

Table 2.3 (Continued)

NMC revalidation requirements		A guide to meeting these requirements
Five reflective accounts	You must record a minimum of five written reflections on CPD and/or a piece of practice-related feedback you have received and/or an event or experience in your own professional practice, and how this relates to the Code.	Each reflection can be about CPD and/or a piece of practice-related feedback you have received and/or an event or experience in your own professional practice, or a combination of all three. For example, an event occurs within your practice, you receive feedback on this, then undertake CPD to support further learning. Your reflective discussion partner and your confirmer will want to see these.
Reflective discussion	You must have a reflective discussion with another NMC registrant covering your five written reflective accounts (see above).	You must ensure that the NMC registrant with whom you had your discussion signs the most up-to-date NMC form recording details such as their name, NMC PIN, email, the date you had the discussion and a summary of the discussion. You must keep this completed form in a safe place. You will be asked to enter these details into NMC Online when you revalidate. Your confirmer will want to see this.
Confirmation	Confirmation involves demonstrating to your confirmer that you have complied with all of the revalidation requirements; it is not about judging your fitness to practise.	Your confirmer will probably be your line manager; they do not have to be an NMC registrant to confirm you. You must ensure your confirmer completes the most up-to-date NMC form recording details such as the name, NMC PIN or other professional identification number (where relevant), email, professional address and postcode of your confirmer. You must keep this completed form in a safe place. You will be asked to enter these details into NMC Online when you revalidate.

(Continued)

Table 2.3 (Continued)

NMC revalidation requirements		A guide to meeting these requirements
Health and character	You must provide a health and character declaration, including any cautions or convictions.	This is a personal declaration only and does not need to be verified by a third party.
Professional indemnity arrangement	You must declare that you have, or will have when practising, appropriate cover under an indemnity arrangement.	If you work for the NHS, they are a member of and covered by the Clinical Negligence and Other Risks Indemnity Scheme (CNORIS). For NHS-employed registrants this is inherent within the organization's vicarious liability for staff. If you are employed by any other organization, please check their indemnity arrangements.
Keeping a portfolio	It is strongly recommended that you keep evidence that you have met the revalidation requirements in a portfolio. This does not necessarily need to be an e-portfolio.	The portfolio will be helpful for the discussion you have with your confirmer. You will also need to have this information available in case the NMC request additional information as part of the verification process (see Chapter 10).

(NMC 2015e)

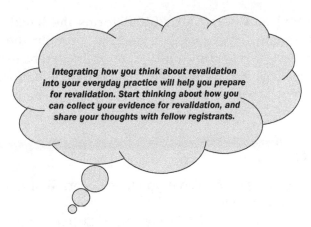

Integrating how you think about revalidation into your everyday practice will help you prepare for revalidation. Start thinking about how you can collect your evidence for revalidation, and share your thoughts with fellow registrants.

Figure 2.4 Are you 'Revalidation Ready'?

Advice/tips for success

✓ I know my revalidation date.
✓ I have registered with NMC Online.
✓ I have checked the NMC website and read the most up-to-date revalidation guidance.
✓ I have started to collate my portfolio of evidence using the required NMC templates.
✓ I know who my reflective discussion partner is.
✓ I know who my confirmer is.
✓ I have spoken to my reflective discussion partner.
✓ I have spoken to my confirmer.
✓ I have encouraged my confirmer and my reflective discussion partner to read the NMC revalidation guidance (NMC 2015e) and confirmer guidance (NMC 2015f).
✓ I have planned a date for my reflective discussion.
✓ I have planned a date for my confirmation discussion.

Overall, revalidation should support nurses and midwives to deliver the best possible care and practice in the most effective way they can (NMC 2015e).

Summary

This chapter has outlined what it means to be a professional and the responsibilities that come with being registered with a regulatory body. The revised Code (NMC 2015a) forms the backbone of the nursing and midwifery profession and has brought the standards expected of every registrant up to date with current expectations and practice. This has formed the basis for revalidation, a simple model which will ensure every registered nurse and midwife is fit for practice.

Key points

- Start preparing now, even if you have a period of time until you are due to revalidate.
- Get familiar with the NMC Code (NMC 2015a).
- Start talking to your colleagues about getting revalidation ready!
- Share ideas with other registrants. Find out what they have completed and how easy it is to revalidate.

CHAPTER

3 Adult learning

This book is designed to help you successfully revalidate, but a key aspect of this is engaging with lifelong learning which has benefits to you as an individual as well as to your practice. This chapter will use different approaches to explore how you learn, with the aim that as you read through you will be able to identify your own learning styles and preferences and identify different types of learning that you could undertake, such as self-directed learning, e-learning, interprofessional learning and more. An overview of the assumptions made about adult learners is described, and the concept of experiential learning and Kolb's Learning Cycle (Kolb 1984) will be explored. This chapter will also explore motivation to learn as well as any barriers you may face, and then proceeds to suggest tools for identifying strengths and weaknesses in relation to learning opportunities (using a SWOT analysis). At the end of the chapter you will find some questions that you can use to help plan your own learning and future CPD activities.

> ### Learning objectives
>
> By the end of the chapter you will be able to:
>
> - Explain the differences between surface, deep and strategic approaches to learning.
> - Explore different learning styles and identify your own preferences.
> - Utilize SWOT analysis to assist with planning your learning.
> - Make a detailed plan in relation to your future learning activities.

Introduction

Learning simply means the acquisition of knowledge or skills through study, experience, or being taught. In actual fact, learning is inevitable – we all learn things, whether we realize it or not, in every day of our life, both personally and professionally. As registrants we have a strong professional obligation to engage in lifelong learning, and the introduction of revalidation simply reinforces this (Kolyva 2015). The way we learn or have been taught has an influence on our preferences. For example, you may have had experiences of going to lectures, when a subject expert speaks at you for a period of time, imparting their knowledge to you. They are the 'font of knowledge' and you are an 'empty vessel' waiting for the knowledge to be poured into your head! This is a very traditional way of learning and can result in superficial learning taking place. According to Biggs (2003), knowledge cannot be imposed in this way; it has to be 'constructed', and this occurs in four ways:

1   Through the development of clear learning objectives.
2   Motivation to learn.
3   Allowing space to learn.
4   Collaborative learning, where discussion with others takes place.

When all of these components exist, then deeper, more meaningful learning can take place. It is therefore important to recognize different approaches to learning.

Approaches to learning

It may be helpful to consider the different approaches you take to learning. These generally fall into one of two categories: either surface learning or deep learning (Entwistle 1981). These terms can be used to describe the approach the individual may use to learn, but are not fixed attributes of the individual; indeed, some individuals may use both approaches for different aspects of learning. An example of surface learning may be a midwife learning about a new medication by memorizing this information. If she could describe to others how this medication works, relate this to her existing knowledge of anatomy and physiology and link this to a rationale for use within this specialty, this would be an example of deeper learning.

If you use a mixture of both deep and surface learning, this is known as strategic learning. This involves learning or performing an educational activity for a defined purpose. You could say that undertaking CPD only to achieve the NMC revalidation guidelines is strategic learning; this has limited benefits if it is only done to achieve your revalidation!

Within both approaches there are specific characteristics and these are defined in Table 3.1.

Deep learning is often the most appropriate approach to learning as this will involve relating what you have learned to developing and influencing your practice. Deep learning often takes more time and effort; however, it is essential for many aspects of your practice. An example could be if you only knew the structure of an eye but, while working in opthalmology, you realized you didn't understand the causes of cataract disease and took the time to study this and find out more. However, if you learn everything deeply this could become very time-consuming. For instance, if you work in cardiology,

Table 3.1 Characteristics of surface and deep learning approaches

Surface	Deep
Tries to predict what learning is necessary in order to plan this.	Combines new knowledge with new learning or combines knowledge from multiple sources.
Information is often memorized and not fully understood.	Assimilates knowledge into an organized structure.
Learning is undertaken to achieve the end result – e.g. passing an exam rather than understanding.	Often evokes enjoyment and a feeling of achieving a challenging activity.
Focus is on achieving the task and can be driven by fear of failure.	Focus comes from the learner.
Information is put together but without the depth of understanding which would occur in deep learning.	Makes sense of information as evidence and formulated arguments.
Information and learning are not related but kept separately. This can lead to learning that does not link elements together and therefore the learning is more superficial than deep learning.	Can link theory and explanation to everyday activities or tasks.

Adapted from Ramsden (1988)

having an in-depth understanding of cataract disease may be useful, but it is not essential to your role. It is therefore a good idea to plan your approach to learning depending on the situation, and this may change over time depending on your scope of practice.

Time Out

Consider something you learned recently where you used a deep learning strategy.

Why did you use this method?

When do you prefer to use surface, deep or strategic learning styles?

We have explored how you may approach learning; now we will consider how you learn. There are many theories about how we learn. This is a subject which has been written about extensively, and if you are interested in reading about this in more depth there are many sources of learning in relation to these theories. You may be familiar with learning by undertaking a task, activity or skill. This is known as experiential learning, which will be explored next.

Experiential learning and Kolb's learning cycle

You may feel you learn a lot simply through things you have experienced, and this can be defined as 'learning through reflection on doing' (Patrick 2011). This has obvious relevance for nursing and midwifery where much of the role is learned through observation of practice, reflection on learning and supervised practice. The pre-registration education of nurses comprises both practical and theoretical components, which very much complements this learning approach. Kolb's experiential learning cycle is a model which encompasses reflection and can be useful when attempting to demystify new knowledge or information (Kolb 1984).

You can work through Kolb's learning cycle on your own, but there are added benefits if you can work through this with a peer or colleague. This has been found to deepen your learning by seeking further feedback and reflection on the event so you can learn from this and improve your practice.

Pause for Thought

Remember: by completing Kolb's learning cycle you would be able to consider any feedback, reflection or any CPD you complete as part of your evidence for revalidation.

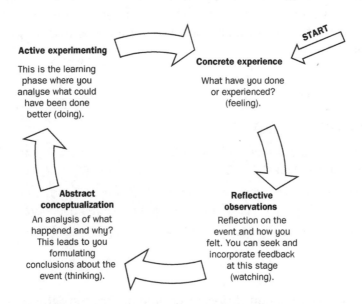

Figure 3.1 Kolb's learning cycle (adapted from Kolb 1984)

Kolb's learning cycle comprises of four parts, starting with 'concrete experience', 'reflective observation', then 'abstract conceptualization' and finally 'active experimentation' – see Figure 3.1. Following Kolb's cycle (1984) in a clockwise direction, each aspect will be discussed.

● Concrete experience (Feeling): Usually the cycle starts with a concrete experience; this means you have done or experienced something, usually an activity or an event.

- Reflective observation (Watching): This encourages you to reflect back on the event or experience and question how you felt and what you felt about the outcome. You may seek feedback at this point.
- Abstract conceptualization (Thinking): This stage encourages you to analyse what happened and come to a conclusion based on your observations. By 'thinking' you will understand more about the event or experience having explored why it occurred in that way.
- Active experimentation (Doing): As the name suggests, this is where you use your learning, make plans or test theories. You might ask yourself how might things have been done differently to achieve another outcome? This phase begins the cycle again as your active experimentation is another new learning experience to explore.

Pause for Thought

What skills or tasks have you undertaken in your practice that were learned experientially?

Were you aware you were following this cycle or did you learn in a different way? Did you seek feedback from others as you learned?

Consider logging any learning you have undertaken as CPD for your revalidation evidence.

Kolb (1984) explains that different people naturally prefer a certain single different learning style; however, various factors can influence a person's preferred style such as the situation, learning activity and time. We will explore learning styles next.

Learning styles

Exploring how you prefer to learn is a key element of successful learning as it can equip you to learn in a way that is natural and fosters your awareness of the areas where you have a preference or dislike. Taking time to understand your learning style means you can undertake learning suited to your style, or perhaps you can make adjustments or plan ways to cope with styles that are less prominent for you.

The types of learning styles were first identified with Honey and Mumford (1986a) and a questionnaire was developed to enable you to work out which learning styles were most prominent within your learning (Honey and Mumford 1986b). If you search the internet you may find links to free websites that you can access to complete the questionnaire. However, you may also recognize your learning style by the descriptions that follow each of the four styles.

1   Activist
2   Pragmatist
3   Theorist
4   Reflector

Each learning style will be discussed with the purpose of encouraging you to recognize your own style and choose learning which suits you best. This can help you choose learning activities that can be recorded as either participatory or individual learning which can be used as CPD for your revalidation evidence.

Activists

These are individuals who live life for today! They enjoy and embrace new experiences which they are motivated to seek out and try. They often act first and think later, which could present problems within a healthcare setting. Activists often enjoy learning that centres on them, so involvement in learning is key.

Examples of learning activities they would normally enjoy include those that contain:

- Brainstorming.
- Problem-solving.
- Group discussions.
- Role play.

Activists are good at – active role	Not so good at – passive role
Games, teamwork.	Assimilation of lots of data.
Excitement, high-energy activities and change.	Reading information by themselves.
Being involved in a key role which may include presentations, leading discussions or study sessions.	Engaging when there is no variance in teaching methods – e.g. teaching using a lecture type format – this induces boredom and disconnection.
Interactive and involvement with others.	Listening to lectures where they are not interactive.

Pragmatists

These individuals need to see the practical relevance to the learning undertaken. Where 'off-the-wall' teaching methods are deployed – e.g. making a collage of views or making models out of paper – they can often disengage unless the relevance is made explicitly. Pragmatists tend to want to make decisions and act on them which can result in frustration where there is a delay. Despite this, they often enjoy experimentation with new theories, practical application and new ideas.

Examples of learning activities they would normally enjoy include those that contain:

● Practical elements.
● Case studies.
● Problem-solving.
● Group discussions.

Pragmatists are good at – active role	Not so good at – passive role
Linking subjects and problems.	Engaging when there is no relevance to current work.
Relevance of techniques to the real world.	Engaging when there is no clear positive outcome.
Can try out new techniques within a safe environment to allow feedback.	Engaging when there are no defined parameters on learning – e.g. no practice guidelines.

Theorists

These individuals are very rational, objective, logical and focused. Theorists enjoy factual information that they can elaborate and develop into theories. Their preference for theory can be seen in their preference to applying principles, theories or development of a model to formulate a rational solution.

Examples of learning activities they would normally enjoy include those that contain:

- Models.
- Statistics.
- Storytelling.
- Tutorials (giving them the lead role).
- Using quotes.

Theorists are good at – active role	Not so good at – passive role
Structured, clear and objective sessions.	Unstructured or not well-defined sessions with minimal direction.
Time to explore theories, models etc. which can include high-level complex problem-solving.	Undertaking alternative experiential techniques that often lead to minimal or surface learning.
Taking part in learning activities where there are mainly right or wrong answers.	Subjects that are not theoretical enough and may be more philosophically based with no defined answers.

Reflectors

These individuals tend to proceed with caution and often consider very carefully their course of action before engaging. Prior to this they may want to connect with others to get different viewpoints and opinions as the way they collect information can either be as an individual or through others. Once information is collected, reflectors may still take time to engage with it as they think deeply about things. Given this, they can often hold back and will assimilate what other are saying and doing before committing themselves to action.

Individuals who are reflectors like learning activities that include those that contain:

- Self-analysis or personality questionnaires.
- Time Out activities.

- Observational activities.
- Feedback from others.
- Paired discussions.
- Coaching or interviews.

Reflectors are good at – active role	Not so good at – passive role
Being left to formulate their own conclusions provided they are given enough time and not pressurized.	Where they are rushed to undertake tasks or make decisions without full consideration.
Active listening and observation from others, or activities or events occurring around them.	Where they are not given enough information or time to prepare.
Taking a less active role or introverted style.	Being forced into an active or extroverted style.

The examples in the tables are designed to assist in identifying which learning style is your preference and support you to adapt strategies to assist if the learning is not your preference. For example, if you were an 'activist' style of learner and you attended a very formal theoretical lecture on home birth you may wish to engage in a tutorial group (or organize your own) to discuss these principles further. Your learning style may evolve over time and is often changed by your experiences (Race 2001).

VARK model

Another simple tool which relates to you identifying your individual learning style is the VARK model (Fleming and Baume 2006). Within this model there is an assumption that we each have a preference to learn through a particular means of delivery, and these are categorized as:

Visual.
Aural or auditory.
Reading or writing.
Kinaesthetic (movement, or doing).

In simple terms, some of us like to learn through seeing, hearing, reading or writing, and others by doing.

Time Out

Consider something you learned recently. Did you prefer learning through:

Seeing?
Hearing?
Reading?
Writing?
Doing?

Reflect on this and plan a learning activity to meet your preferences. Discuss this with your peers; do they like to learn in the same way?

Types of learning

Once you have identified how you prefer to learn you will want to consider different types of learning you may want to undertake. The main ones are self-directed learning, e-learning, distance learning, interprofessional learning and work-based learning. We are now going to explore each of these in turn.

Self-directed learning

Self-directed learning is where an individual is responsible for selecting, managing and assessing their own learning. It can be undertaken at a place or time that is suitable to them, and can involve different levels of study. For revalidation purposes this is classed as individual learning, unless you undertake this with others.

Pause for Thought

Think about how self-directed you consider yourself to be? Reading this book can be seen as being motivated and self-directed!

When considering self-directed learning, you may want to think about different aspects of learning – both intellectual and practical or physical. Consider the following areas of learning which have been defined by Glazzard et al. (2014):

1   Knowledge: this can be tested by using your memory to recall, and can be tested through oral or written communication – e.g. signs and symptoms of a wound infection.
2   Motor skills: these can be 'taught' but must be independently learned – e.g. correct injection technique.
3   Attitudes and behaviour: these can be learned through role modelling or passed on through demonstration – e.g. exhibiting professional behaviour as a registered nurse or midwife in dealing with relatives' enquires.
4   Intellectual skills: this includes high-level thinking to analyse situations and problem-solve, and may involve adapting how you act as you apply knowledge to different situations – e.g. dealing with a patient who has been diagnosed with depression will involve assessment and analysing their presentation, followed by a plan of action with other healthcare professionals. It will essentially involve multiple skills being adapted to problem-solve and promote patient well-being.

All of the above areas may be those you want to work on via your own self-directed learning. A common type of self-directed learning is e-learning.

e-Learning

Electronic learning is often referred to as 'e-learning', which is learning that can be accessed by computer, tablet or Smartphone. It can comprise of modules given to you to complete as mandatory training as part of your job, or it could involve online seminars or education sessions that can be part of a course or a one-off event.

Time Out

Have you used e-learning previously?

What was this for?

What did you think about your experience of e-learning?

Historically, e-learning has not always been a useful experience due to either the topic or the simplistic design of the learning platform, and this can lead to surface learning. However, this is an area where there have been recent developments which can make the available learning interactive and engaging. Advantages include:

● It can be undertaken at your own pace.
● It can be undertaken at a time suitable to you – this can be useful if you are on shifts and cannot attend formal education during the day.
● You can direct the education, stop at any point and return – therefore it can fit in with your other commitments.
● It can reduce your costs as you do not need to travel or print materials (although you still may wish to do so). This can also have time-management benefits.
● Completion is recorded, often automatically. This can allow you to easily save evidence of completion for revalidation purposes.
● Is often inexpensive or free.

It is important that you find different ways of learning that are meaningful to you so keep an open mind! E-learning is often not available or suitable for all topics as practical elements require detailed graphics and, in some cases, expensive development to make them useful. Some topics allow the theory via e-learning and then a practical element to practise and develop the skills – e.g. cardiopulmonary resuscitation (CPR). Where this is incorporated with another method of learning – e.g. face-to-face learning – it is known as 'blended learning'. You may also have heard of distance learning which often has on online component to it, and this is explored next.

Distance learning

Not all learning has to be undertaken through physical attendance at a course or study day. You may experience learning that involves some form of remote learning which is not through the traditional method of face-to-face teaching; this is often referred to as 'distance learning'. Advances in IT have resulted in many online courses which can be easily accessed and can be free of charge in some instances. This has the key advantage that they can be undertaken in any location at any time. If considering this option, ensure that the teaching materials come from a source that is credible and best suited to your needs. Also consider your learning style; if you are an activist, for example, this style of learning may not always suit you. In the case of undertaking a structured course, online discussions and tutorials with peers may comprise a key component of the course content. The Open University is probably the most popular and well-established organization to offer undergraduate and other courses through a flexible learning approach.

Within healthcare we often learn with other professionals either due to them being accessible in practice – for instance, learning informally together in the clinical area or where both parties have the same learning need in a formal setting, e.g. physiotherapists and nurses both learning about asthma medication on an accredited course. This leads to interprofessional learning, which will be explored next.

Interprofessional learning

Interprofessional learning has been described as education:

> 'that occurs when two or more professions learn with, from and about each other to improve collaboration and the quality of care'.

> (CAIPE 2002)

Time Out

Think of an example of a time when you have been involved in interprofessional learning – e.g. multiprofessional ward rounds, team meetings, incident investigations or formalized courses.

What were the advantages in involving other professionals in your learning?

Did this have a positive outcome? If not, why not?

Remember that any new ways of working, such as interprofessional learning, may have hurdles that are worth persevering with. Buring et al. (2009) cite the main barriers to interprofessional learning as those relating to logistical and resource issues, and they suggest that planning is a key element for success.

Pause for Thought

Consider interprofessional learning as an opportunity to share experiences of preparing for revalidation.

Interprofessional learning is participatory, as you are learning with others, and can be used as evidence of CPD for revalidation purposes (see Chapter 4). You do not have to learn with another NMC registrant; in fact, often you can learn more from your wider team (NMC 2015e). This type of learning usually occurs within practice and therefore could also be defined as 'work-based learning'.

Work-based learning

Work-based learning is a good way to enhance your career and employment prospects while gaining learning or qualifications without having to study full-time. It can take a number of guises, from informal teaching sessions to formal qualifications; however, this is often the type of learning that happens informally every day within practice. For example, a child may ask you to explain why they have been given this treatment, and by explaining this to them using language they understand you will hopefully have learned something, which might be a good communication technique, or perhaps prompt you to research the child's condition in more depth.

This type of learning is well suited to nursing and midwifery as it is often a highly practical profession and, in conjunction with a work-based mentor, it can be a good way to ensure successful learning. Often when implementing formal work-based learning within a job role a contract may be drawn up, known as a learning contract. This ensures that expectations from both parties are met and defines the responsibilities of both. Activities relating to work-based learning are explored in more detail in Chapter 4.

SWOT analysis

You may have heard of a SWOT analysis (MindTools.com 2016). SWOT stands for Strengths, Weaknesses, Opportunities and Threats. The strengths and weaknesses are internal and the opportunities and threats are external. This is a valuable tool which can help you understand how you or your team can make positive changes by assessing either your individual learning needs or those within a team. This could show gaps within a department or service which could be potentially problematic if not addressed; thus it assists in planning for the future or analysing a problem. This can be useful for you as it will help to define learning activities you may undertake, which can be used for revalidation purposes.

For each quadrant heading, ask yourself the following:

Strengths – what is working well?
Weaknesses – what needs improvement or change?
Opportunities – what opportunities are around us?
Threats – what obstacles do we face?

Strengths	Opportunities
Prompts	Prompts
• What am I/the team good at, or what skills or knowledge do the team have? • What benefits can be identified? • Does this relate to skills or knowledge? • What are the key achievements? • Does this relate to a specific skill?	• What possible plans are available that could be beneficial? • What is new and could be utilized for the benefit of yourself or the team? • What is happening that could help me or the team? • In terms of learning, is the course run in-house (no cost) or external with funding available?
Weaknesses	Threats
Prompts	Prompts
• What could you improve? • What should you avoid? • What do people in your team feel are the weaknesses, or what do you see as weaknesses?	• What individuals or actions could compromise what I or the team want to achieve? • What are the threats if this issue is not addressed? • What could threaten our success?

Time Out

Consider completing your own SWOT analysis. In order to undertake this activity, ensure you have time to dedicate to the task and, if undertaking this as part of a team, set ground rules and give clear instructions.

Draw a large square (if doing this as a team a whiteboard or flip chart is ideal). Divide the square into quadrants and label strengths, weaknesses, opportunities and threats.

After completion of the quadrants you can analyse the results which should help to show where you need to focus to achieve your goals when planning your learning. Try to make plans to achieve this and note aspects that you did not expect. Consider the four questions below when planning for success.

1   How can the strengths be further developed and extended?
2   How can the weaknesses be managed to reduce their impact and, if possible, be overcome?
3   How can the opportunities be harnessed for maximum impact?
4   How can the threats be reduced or avoided? This could involve better planning, discussion with management, etc.

The example shown in Table 3.2 illustrates where you could use a SWOT analysis to plan the learning needs of a service or team.

The results of undertaking this SWOT analysis was that measures were taken to release staff to undertake the training, and that this needed to be planned. In addition, a mentoring role was also introduced to support staff in practice, after a discussion that this would be helpful to link theory to practical 'hands-on' experiences.

Utilizing the SWOT analysis could be a useful tool when planning the educational needs for a team or department and show the deficits as well as strengths. Your own behaviour and attitude has a key role to play in both your own learning and that of others.

Table 3.2 SWOT analysis of the need for advanced life support skills within an accident and emergency department

Strengths	Opportunities
Most staff have undertaken advanced life support training. This results in the resuscitation room always having a qualified member of staff available to deal with emergencies.	Advanced life support courses are run twice a year. Many staff within the unit have completed the course leading to a good skill base relating to applying theory to practice in advanced life support skills. This could mean that additional staff who undertake the course could have an in-house mentor within the department.

Weaknesses	Threats
With staff turnover and sickness levels the number of staff with this skill has reduced over the past three months. This could potentially result in no staff member being on duty who has undertaken the course and/or had recent experience of using this skill. Course is three days out of the clinical environment.	If staffing levels were poor, agency staff who come to the unit do not have advanced life support training. Thus, only permanent staff can work in the resuscitation room. This could result in not having a member of staff on duty with advanced life support training, leading to a risk for patients. If a staff member had recently completed the course, would they have the experience to deal with all situations? After discussion, this was something that could not be guaranteed, stressing the importance of practical experience.

Adult learning

Malcolm Knowles was a leader within the theory of adult learning and described six key assumptions about adult learners. These 'assumptions' relate to the aspects surrounding successful adult learning and are discussed next.

Six assumptions of adult learners (based on Knowles et al. 2005).

1   **Need to know:** We want to know why we need to learn something before undertaking learning.
2   **Learners' self-concept:** This is how we view ourselves, similar to self-awareness. We believe we are responsible for

our lives; we need to be seen and treated as capable and self-directed.

3   **Learners' experience:** We all come with different experiences. There are individual differences in background, learning style, motivation, needs, interests, and goals, creating a greater need for individualization of learning strategies (Brookfield 1986; Silberman and Auerbach 1998). The richest resource for learning resides in you; tapping into your experiences through experiential techniques (discussions, simulations, problem-solving activities, or case methods) is beneficial (Brookfield 1986; Silberman and Auerbach 1998; McKeachie 2002; Knowles et al. 2005).

4   **Readiness to learn:** We become ready to learn things we need to know and do in order to cope effectively with real-life situations. We want to learn what we can apply in the present, making learning activities that are focused on the future or that do not relate to our current situation less effective.

5   **Orientation to learning:** We are life-centred in our orientation to learning. We want to learn what will help us perform tasks or deal with problems we confront in everyday situations and those presented in the context of application to real life (Merriam and Caffarella 1999).

6   **Motivation to learn:** We are responsive to some external motivators (e.g. better job, higher salary), but the most potent motivators are internal (e.g. desire for increased job satisfaction, self-esteem). Motivation can be blocked by education that ignores these adult learning principles.

Time Out

Reflect on your own learning experiences. Can you identify with any of Knowles' assumptions of adult learners?

Motivation

Consider what you have read about how adults learn. It is easy to see that motivation is key to successful learning. This can be broken into two aspects: intrinsic and extrinsic motivation.

Intrinsic motivation is where you engage in a learning activity for its own sake because you find it enjoyable. For example:

● Self-satisfaction – you simply enjoy the activity.
● Feeling valued.
● Engagement with topics and educational activities that you have chosen and had control over.
● Stimulating.

An example of this would be an interest in palliative care which resulted in attendance at a study event. You are therefore motivated to attend this study event because the topic interests you.

Extrinsic motivation is where you are driven to learn by factors external to you. For example:

● Expectations of others.
● Your employer or your regulator.
● Reward or praise.
● Your colleagues.

An example of this would be child protection training which is mandatory within your job description as a health visitor and failure to comply would result in you being unable to fulfil your role. You are therefore motivated to complete this to meet your employer's requirements.

Your motivation can change depending on a number of factors, and are time and context dependent. For example, you may be motivated to complete your e-learning because you have a deadline to meet. You may choose to read about a topic such as telehealth because it interests you, but you lose motivation because you don't want to do this in your own time.

Time Out

Think about the last study session/event you attended or article you read.
What motivated you to undertake this learning?

Was this an area of interest, part of your personal development plan (PDP) or personal interest?

Compare this to your experience of undertaking mandatory or compulsory training.

Were they both enjoyable and stimulating? If not, why not?

Consider your intrinsic and extrinsic motivation for undertaking each type of learning activity.

Remember: you can log this Time Out activity as evidence of individual CPD and use this towards meeting your revalidation requirements.

In each case you could compare different factors such as the topic area, methods of delivery of the information or training, and the end result of the educational activity (registered qualification, application to practice etc.).

In the Time Out activity, you may have reflected on the following points:

- Did you undertake learning that was relevant? This may include practical knowledge in relation to your role – for example, a specific area like venepuncture or cannulation.
- Were the educational sessions successful and did they fulfil your desire to undertake this skill? In some instances, they may correlate with immediate benefits for patients – e.g. being able to undertake venepucture on a patient instead of waiting for the phlebotomist or another staff member to be free to undertake this.
- Were innovative learning approaches utilized? Utilizing innovative learning approaches was explored earlier in relation to styles of learning, but approaches may include: podcasts, videos, online learning, using WebEx, discussions with colleagues, journal clubs, participation in a community of practice, etc. These 'new' ways of learning may keep your interest by appealing to a visual or experiential way of learning, or suggest new ways of learning that you have not previously undertaken.
- Were you able to keep up with the speed of learning, or was it too slow? Undertaking education or learning at your own speed

is important because if it goes too fast you may become overwhelmed. But if it is too slow, it may become dull and boring,
leading to a lack of concentration. Timing is also crucial – trying
to assimilate knowledge after a night shift is perhaps not the
best choice!

- Did it engage your heart and mind? Using your personal life and
  work experiences to guide your interest and motivation to learn
  has clear benefits to keeping your interest and expanding your
  knowledge base in the topic too.
- When you undertook the learning, did you have a good grasp of
  the benefits it would bring to you and your practice? Will the
  learning be for revalidation, your PDP, an award or certificate,
  or a mixture of these?

Barriers to learning

You may feel that there are barriers to your learning. The following
list provides a very negative list of characteristics, which when
assembled together appear to describe a very unmotivated learner.
However, barriers to learning may be experienced by anyone at any
time, and you might be better encouraged to recognize these as an
overview, rather than absolute categories.

- Lack of confidence.
- Low or uncertain motivation.
- Inattentiveness or lack of attendance/participation.
- Poor listening skills.
- Underdeveloped study skills.
- Anxiety, fear or insecurity.
- Incomplete prior knowledge.
- Previous experience of failure/difficulty in learning.
- Domestic, financial or personal worries.
- Low expectations of self.
- Unrealistic expectations of self.
- Unwillingness to ask for help.
- Physical or health conditions.
- Mental health conditions.
- Specific learning difficulties, etc.

Pause for Thought

When considering some of these barriers, you should reflect on your learning style to overcome these. For example, if you lack motivation then you should, where possible, select a learning activity in a style which does motivate you   e.g. using a mind map to develop your knowledge on a particular topic instead of making a list.

Planning your learning

Primarily you need to assess what you need or want to learn and what your position is in relation to this (see also Chapter 4). This is sometimes referred to as a 'gap' in knowledge, skills or practice. You may identify this as part of your appraisal, feedback from others (including colleagues, patients or service users), undertaking a new job role or a personal interest. This may also have been undertaken in your individual or team SWOT analysis. Table 3.3 shows the difference between knowledge, skills and practice and gives some examples relating to staff nurse Bani Singh, who has just started a new post in a gastrointestinal unit.

It is important to discuss your learning needs with your manager to secure support which, in some instances, can include funding, time

Table 3.3 Identifying learning needs

Type	Definition	Example
Knowledge	Understanding of principles or aspects of new clinical practice.	Deficit in knowledge of common gastrointestinal disorder and treatments following successful appointment to this new area of practice.
Skills	The ability to undertake an activity or relate procedural knowledge.	The ability to perform nasogastric tube aspiration.
Practice	The ability to successfully apply or demonstrate knowledge or skills in practice.	Be able to plan care for a patient with a specific gastrointestinal disorder using knowledge and skills.

away from work to attend, help in securing supervised practice or the need for a work-based mentor. This can be included in your personal development plan, and the following questions may be useful to consider:

- Why is this training or education necessary? A strong personal and work rationale will put your learning needs high on your manager's agenda.
- Why undertake it now? Does your timescale and that of your employer match? This will be key if it is necessary to be released from work for the educational session – e.g. if this is being held during the peak holiday time then it may not be ideal.
- What relevance and interest is the topic to me, my working environment, future career aspirations? Where your interest and work aligns there is a high chance of success for both parties. This may include personal development – e.g. leadership courses where this will develop your role now and in the future.
- What will the outcome of the learning be? Will you be required to sit an exam or undertake supervised practice? Is it formal or informal? What commitment does it involve – time, money or resources? If this is a formal qualification – e.g. a Masters in Education for a future role in education, the contribution in terms of time off work and course fees can vary depending on your employer.
- What options are available to achieve this? Consider varied ways of learning depending on the topic – e.g. shadowing, internal or external study sessions by subject experts, reading relevant journals or books. (See also Chapter 4 on CPD which can help you to identify suitable activities for your development).
- How are you going to evidence and record your learning? This is essential as evidence for revalidation, and Chapter 10 provides further information regarding developing your portfolio of evidence.

Once you have identified your learning needs it is important to make a plan of how you will achieve the learning you have set out to do. You can use the CPD planner tool in Chapter 4 to help you.

Summary

Professional development is all about continuous learning and education so that you, as a nurse or midwife, can provide the very best care to the service users, patients and families that you engage with professionally. Finding out how you learn and what your preferences are is very powerful and will help you to achieve your goals. However, your professional development should also be planned, systematic and managed in such a way as to ensure that you always have the current knowledge and skills necessary to practise in a safe, caring and effective way. This chapter has explored adult learning in general, considering your preferences, team needs and learning styles. The next chapter will focus more specifically on CPD with the objective of helping you identify CPD activities you could complete for use in the revalidation process and to support developments in your knowledge and skills.

Key points

- Lifelong learning is a fundamental part of being a registered professional and can be described as learning throughout your career where you are continually looking to develop and improve your practice.
- Everyone is an individual learner, and the approaches and styles you prefer may not suit someone else. Be aware of this when learning as part of a group.
- There are many learning opportunities around you in practice. Seek these out and be adventurous!

Continuing professional development (CPD)

Introduction

Every registered nurse and midwife has a responsibility to keep their professional knowledge and skills up to date with practice throughout their career. One of the ways this can be achieved is through continuing professional development, which is often referred to as CPD. This chapter will explore the different ways in which CPD can be undertaken across a variety of roles, as well as equip you to identify your learning needs and plan CPD activities for revalidation.

Learning objectives

By the end of this chapter you will be able to:

- Self-assess your CPD learning needs.
- Identify CPD activities that will enable you to develop your practice.
- Develop a plan of appropriate CPD activities relevant to your scope of practice.
- Address barriers to completion of your CPD.

Current NMC revalidation requirements

The NMC (2015e: 16) states that:

'You must undertake 35 hours of continuing professional development (CPD) relevant to your scope of practice as a nurse or midwife, over the three years prior to the renewal of your registration. Of those 35 hours of CPD, 20 must include participatory learning.'

Always refer to the NMC website for the most up-to-date revalidation guidance.

These are the minimum hours set by the NMC; however, it is in your best interest to undertake as much CPD as is necessary for you to keep your knowledge and skills up to date. It is important that you clearly demonstrate how you have developed and what has changed as a result of any learning you undertake. You are responsible for your own continuing professional development; if you work for an organization they may support you with this, but the responsibility to complete this learning lies with you. As a professional you have a duty to keep your knowledge and skills up to date.

CPD records

Your CPD records can be held in many different ways, but using the key requirements from the NMC listed below as headings is a good place to start. Keep these in mind whenever you are planning CPD activities.

The NMC key requirements are that you must keep a record of:

- Dates the CPD activity was undertaken.
- CPD method – e.g. online learning, face-to-face study day, interactive workshop.
- A brief description of the topic and how it relates to your practice.
- Identification of the part(s) of the Code (NMC 2015a) most relevant to the CPD.
- Number of hours and participatory hours.
- Evidence of the CPD activity.

(NMC 2015e)

The Code: Professional Standards of Practice and Behaviour for Nurses and Midwives (NMC 2015a: 7) Section 6 explains the standard required of every registrant in relation to CPD:

6. Always practise in line with the best available evidence.

6.1 Make sure that any information or advice given is evidence-based, including information relating to using any healthcare products or services, and

6.2 Maintain the knowledge and skills you need for safe and effective practice.

NMC CPD requirements

The NMC do not prescribe which CPD activities you should undertake, but they must relate to your scope of practice. The NMC guidance suggests that mandatory training, such as fire safety or health and safety, which does not directly relate to your scope of practice, may not count as CPD. Other training, such as basic life support or equality and diversity training, may count if it is relevant to your role (NMC 2015e). If you are in any doubt as to what can be counted towards your CPD hours then it is advisable to speak to your confirmer at the earliest opportunity. (For information on confirmers, see Chapter 8.)

Definition of CPD

CPD stands for continuing professional development, which is the learning you undertake as part of your ongoing professional development. This should be a continuous process of learning and reflection used to keep up to date or to develop new knowledge and skills; it is not simply about undertaking training. CPD can involve any relevant learning activity, whether formal and struc-tured or informal and self-directed (we cover self-directed learning in more detail in the next section). CPD provides assurance to the public by ensuring that registrants uphold professional standards through the maintenance of professional competence. CPD has been defined as: 'The maintenance and enhancement of the knowl-edge, expertise and competence of professionals throughout their careers according to a plan formulated with regard to the needs of the professional, the employer, the profession and society' (Madden and Mitchell 1993: 12).

The purpose of CPD is to keep your knowledge and skills up to date, to ensure you can practise safely, and is often referred to as lifelong learning (also covered in Chapter 3). CPD can also have benefits such as career development or promotion due to the development of additional knowledge and skills (Smith and Desai 2010). Within your day-to-day practice you learn continuously, often without consciously realizing it, and often this is not logged anywhere. It is important to record your CPD as it allows you to recognize changes to your practice as they occur, helps track your own development, and demonstrates your commitment to ongoing professional development.

Individual learning

Individual learning simply means learning on your own. This may take place in a variety of settings and can happen during a working day or at any time using a Smartphone or computer (see Table 4.1 for examples). There are limitations to this approach, including the inability to discuss your learning with others, but there are also benefits because you are responsible for developing and shaping your own learning goals and achievements. For some registrants who work in isolation, individual learning may be a common event. It is important to take every opportunity you can to learn, and remember that to meet the NMC revalidation requirements you must also take part in participatory learning. There is no requirement to complete any individual learning to meet the requirements for revalidation, but most registrants will have

Table 4.1 Types of individual learning activities

Learning activity	Examples of CPD
Self-directed learning (directed private study)	Completing activities from this book! Reading books or journal articles. Completing a workbook or reading. Notes/handouts. Watching pre-recorded presentations or video clips.
Online learning	Researching or reading articles on the internet. eLearning modules. RSS (Really Simple Syndicate) Feeds (see later in the chapter). Podcasts or WebEx.
Distance learning	Formal courses often hosted online provided by higher education institutions, such as a degree course or Masters modules.

evidence of this – i.e. all 35 hours can be participatory, but not all 35 can be self-directed – 20 of these must be participatory.

Participatory learning

Individual and participatory learning are equally important. CPD should keep you up to date and competent within your scope of practice as well as supporting changes in your practice. This can be achieved by participating in a learning activity with any other member of your team or with patients or service users (see Table 4.2). Interprofessional learning is equally important and also counts as CPD, and can be done with another registrant or another member of your team to count as participatory. They do not have to be registered with the NMC, and you may engage with other professionals who are not healthcare professionals – for example, students, social workers, receptionists, portering staff etc. (see also Chapter 3).

Share your skills! If you work in isolation as a sole practitioner you may find it beneficial to organize a peer group where you can share learning from each other's CPD or use this group to facilitate CPD activities. However, the deepest learning is achieved when you learn with others, and the ability to discuss and challenge what you have gained and how it has influenced your practice is an important step in your professional development (Quinn 1998).

Table 4.2 Types of participatory learning activities

Learning activity	Examples of CPD
Work-based learning	Learning by doing.
	Shadowing.
	Coaching.
	Mentorship.
	Clinical skills.
Professional activity	Giving a presentation at a conference.
	Teaching a colleague.
	Writing an article for publication.
	Seminars.
	Conferences.
	Workshops.
	Study days.

Table 4.2 (Continued)

Learning activity	Examples of CPD
Formal education	Training course. Further education. Short courses.
Informal education	Discussing practice/patient care. Discussing evidence-based practice. Informal teaching sessions. Blogs. Social media.

Pause for Thought

Discuss with your colleagues what CPD activities they have undertaken in the last year. This may give you some ideas you hadn't thought of.

Opportunities

Many of us ask ourselves 'Where do I begin?', and identifying opportunities for CPD can sometimes cause difficulties, particularly when formal education isn't possible. Study days or course attendance remains one of the most popular methods of CPD, but with the availability of the internet and online resources increasing there is an opportunity to be more creative. Not all CPD activities will be planned; opportunities may arise within your everyday practice for informal learning to take place. This can often be the most valuable form of CPD because it relates to your everyday practice – for example, preparing a session plan for a teaching session as part of your day-to-day practice is CPD providing you have learned something, applied this to your practice, and can link it to the Code (NMC 2015a). However, it is important for you to identify when this learning has taken place so you can take time to reflect on this 'unplanned' CPD and consider the wider implications, including the impact, expected benefits to your practice and links to the Code (NMC 2015a).

Self-assessment tool

A self-assessment tool can be used to help identify your learning needs. The tool below contains a series of questions that can help to focus you as you identify and plan CPD activities. You may also wish to use the tool in Box 4.1 to guide your appraisal or reflective conversation (for more on these, see Chapter 7).

Box 4.1 Self-assessment tool for appraisal or reflective conversations

Self-assessment tool

- What are my areas of strength?
- Where do I require some development?
- What interests me the most?
- What are my colleagues doing?
- What formal courses do I want to undertake?
- What is already happening within my clinical area that I can access? This may be through another professional group of staff, such as pharmacy or medical staff.

The most important aspect of CPD is that you can relate your learning to your own scope of practice and the Code.

(NMC 2015a)

Barriers to CPD

Time Out

Consider the main barriers to CPD, which are likely to include issues around time management, funding or planning.

Do any of these sound familiar?

How could you overcome these?

The main barrier for many is a lack of time, although other barriers include costs and access. Motivation can also be a factor when planning your CPD; if you lack the motivation to actively seek out learning opportunities then this can also hinder you. A high workload can also make the completion of CPD difficult, particularly if you plan to be released from practice to attend a course or undertake work-based learning.

Time management

It can be challenging to find time to not only complete CPD but also to record it. To meet the minimum requirement of 35 hours over three years, this averages at approximately one hour of CPD per month, and it shouldn't take longer than ten minutes to complete a record of each hour. You may want to set aside this time every month, or you may decide to simply log everything as it happens. Whichever method you decide on, the important aspect is to record the CPD as soon as possible, otherwise you may forget what you did learn or simply forget to log it completely!

Other barriers such as costs, access and motivation can be overcome by realizing that CPD can be part of your everyday practice and, for the most part, shouldn't take extra effort or cost to complete. A lot of CPD can be undertaken without actively planning or having to really think about it. See the CPD tips in Box 4.2.

Funding

If you are looking for funding to support your CPD it is important that you liaise with any internal educational department you may have and further education institutions. They may be able to advise you as to which opportunities are available. Examples of funding to undertake formal education or shadowing are available via organizations such as the Royal College of Nursing, Florence Nightingale Foundation and the Queen's Nursing Institute. Perhaps also consider if you can learn what you want to achieve through a different route – for example, planning a work-based learning activity instead (see Chapter 3).

Box 4.2 CPD tips

- Make a plan of the CPD activities you plan to undertake.
- Rank these in order of priority.
- Decide on when you will complete the activity.
- Break activities down, if possible, into smaller chunks.
- Try and stick to your plan.
- Use simple tools to track your CPD activities (see the NMC website for the most up-to-date templates).

Planning CPD

A CPD activity may arise from different things, such as an incident, query, professional discussion, conversation with a patient, future career planning, mentorship or coaching. When you plan your CPD keep in mind that you are likely to gain the most from the activities that take place in your workplace and are defined as work-based learning.

There are three simple steps to follow:

1   Plan
2   Do
3   Reflect

These do not necessarily have to be followed in that order, as shown in Figure 4.1.

Plan – this may be where you begin, depending on your learning style (see Chapter 3), or you may use this step to plan further development due to a CPD activity you have already completed.
Do – this can be a second step or you may start here if you have perhaps completed some 'unplanned' CPD.
Reflect – this can be the third step or you may find this is where you start, depending on your learning style (see Chapter 3).

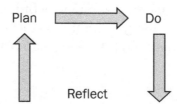

Figure 4.1 Plan: Do: Reflect

You should be able to plan your CPD activities annually with the support of your manager. This often takes place at your annual appraisal, where you meet with your line manager to plan your development activities for the year ahead. When you plan your CPD activities they need to be achievable and positively framed. They should encourage you to complete a set objective – for example: 'complete a practice-based observational audit of handwashing'.

You may have a personal development plan in place, but may find that other learning needs arise throughout the year or even across a day or a week. Support from others is vital to succeed as it helps to encourage and motivate you (see Chapter 8 supportive relationships).

Possible questions you may ask yourself may be:

● Where do I want to be?
● What would I like to know more about?
● What interests me the most?

You may want to set simple short-, medium- and long-term goals, and so a concise to-do list may be all you need! Alternatively, if you prefer a more detailed template you can use the CPD planner tool in Box 4.3 to plan your learning. You can complete this planner either on paper or electronically. Use whichever format you are comfortable with, recognizing the limitations in each approach.

Box 4.3 CPD planner tool

● Identified learning need.
● Learning objectives.
● Possible activities.
● People to speak to and support.
● Priority – high, medium, low.
● Planned activities.
● Planned start and completion dates.
● How will I know I have achieved this learning?

Example of a completed CPD planner tool:

Table 4.3 Completed CPD Planner Tool

Identified learning need	Update knowledge of evidence-based treatments for urinary catheter-related infections.
Learning objectives	Be able to:
	1. Define the criteria used to diagnose a urinary catheter-related infection.
	2. Describe the most appropriate treatment for a urinary catheter-related infection.
	3. Discuss the advantages and disadvantages of current treatments available.

(Continued)

Table 4.3 (Continued)

Possible activities	E-learning, face-to-face course, literature search, policy reading, higher education module, shadow urologist and/or microbiologist, speak to urology nurse specialist and/or infection control team.
People to speak to and support	Senior nurse, line manager, colleagues, local practice education/training and development department, university, urologist, specialist nurses, ward, department.
Priority – high, medium, low	High, due to increased number of patients receiving treatment for urinary catheter-related infections.
Planned activities	Speak to urology nurse specialist/infection control team and complete the relevant eLearning module.
Planned start and completion dates	Start this month (March) to be completed by the end of this month – 31 March.
How will I know I have achieved this learning?	Evidence of completion of the relevant eLearning module. Sharing this learning with colleagues at our team meeting. Reflection on the learning I have undertaken and how I have improved practice as a result.

Setting learning objectives and goals

It can be helpful to use the mnemonic acronym 'SMART' to help guide you when setting learning objectives or goals. It can be difficult to set goals or to understand how you will achieve them. The SMART criteria can be used to make sure you stay on track! See Table 4.4.

Organizing your CPD

The activities you undertake must link to at least one of the four areas of the Code (NMC 2015a). Linking simply means reviewing your learning activity and deciding which section of the Code this relates to. This will also help you to become more familiar with the Code. It is for you to decide what activities you need to undertake; these should cover areas of your practice that you are competent in, as well as areas requiring development. It is recommended that you ensure your CPD covers each of the four areas of the Code, and

Table 4.4 SMART criteria (Adapted from Doran 1981)

S – specific	A specific goal will usually answer the five 'W' questions: • What: What do I want to accomplish? • Why: Specific reasons, purpose or benefits of accomplishing the goal. • Who: Who is involved? • Where: Identify a location. • Which: Identify requirements and constraints.
M – measurable	A measurable goal will usually answer questions such as: • How much? • How many? • How will I know when it is accomplished?
A – achievable	An achievable goal will usually answer the question 'How?': • How can the goal be accomplished? • How realistic is the goal, based on other constraints?
R – realistic	A realistic goal can answer yes to these questions: • Does this seem worthwhile? • Is this the right time? • Does this match my needs? • Are you the right person?
T – time-bound	A time-bound goal will usually answer the question: • When? • What can I do six months from now? • What can I do six weeks from now? • What can I do today?

each activity may link to more than one section. Organizing your portfolio of evidence is covered in Chapter 10.

Four sections of the Code (NMC 2015a):

1   Prioritize People – this section describes standards in relation to preserving dignity and respecting individual needs.
2   Practise Effectively – this section describes standards in relation to evidence-based practice, communication and feedback.
3   Preserve Safety – this section describes standards in relation to working within the limits of your competence and escalating concerns.
4   Promote Professionalism and Trust – this section describes standards in relation to professionalism and standards of conduct and behaviour expected.

You may, for example, select 'Practise Effectively', because you feel this is an area that requires development, and plan an activity related to this section of the Code (NMC 2015a). Continuing the example, you decide to complete an online module on enhanced communication skills and log this as individual CPD. If you then discussed your learning with colleagues, this additional time could also count as participatory CPD.

Time Out

Reflect on your last week at work. What have you learned?

Identify any interactions you had that led to developments within your practice. This may include team meetings, clinical supervision, working with students or looking up evidence-based practice within a journal.

Record your learning using the following headings (NMC 2015e).

- Dates the CPD activity was undertaken.
- CPD method – e.g. online learning, study day.
- A brief description of the topic and how it relates to your practice.
- Identification of the part(s) of the Code (NMC 2015a) most relevant to the CPD.
- Number of hours and participatory hours.
- Evidence of the CPD activity.

Always check the NMC website for the most up-to-date templates.

Recording CPD

Remember to reflect on your learning and link it to the Code (NMC 2015a). Be honest if you don't achieve what you set out to do; you may find you have learned something different to what you expected – that is OK! You may not have learned as much as expected; reflect on this and plan another activity. You should use the most up-to-date template provided by the NMC to record your learning (NMC 2015e).

Top tips

- Try to record your CPD as soon as possible after you have completed it.
- Keep a record of key learning in bullet point format. If you are short of time you can return and complete a fuller record later.
- Use an audio recording that can be typed up if this suits your learning style and is helpful.
- You may want to keep a regular diary or online blog.

Maintaining knowledge and skills

Pause for Thought

Think back to a recent situation you found challenging – can you use CPD to develop your knowledge or skills?

For some reason you may find that you are not at work for a period of time. This may be due to sickness, maternity leave or a career break. It is important you maintain your knowledge and skills within your scope of practice during this time, wherever possible. Most learning is completed within the scope of your role during day-to-day practice; however, to meet revalidation requirements you may have to undertake learning at home or in your own time.

Keeping up to date

Most journals can be accessed online by doing a literature search, and depending on which organization you work for these may be provided free of charge through your library or knowledge services. You can access a number of search engines and databases through OpenAthens, an access management system which simplifies access to a number of electronic resources and journals your organization has subscribed to. Once you have logged into your Open Athens online account you can access and print journal articles.

This service is available free of charge to the majority of registrants working in the NHS and to those organizations providing NHS services. You may not have access to this service or you may choose to pay for an individual subscription to a professional journal instead. Using free search engines such as Google, Yahoo, Bing and Wikipedia should be done with the utmost care as information contained on some websites may not be validated.

Common search engines that can be used for literature searches:

Ovid (Medline, Embase, AMED, HMIC, PsycINFO)
ProQuest (British Nursing Index)
EBSCO (Health Business Elite)
PubMed
Cinahl
BMJ and AMA
Cochrane Library
Dynamed
Nursing Reference Centre Plus
Google Scholar

RSS feeds

RSS stands for Really Simple Syndicate – a way of keeping up to date with the latest information on a website. It saves time by not having to visit each website regularly because you are emailed headlines on a regular basis based on your interests. Most websites indicate the existence of the feed on the home page or main news page with a link to RSS, or sometimes by displaying an orange button with the letters XML or RSS.

Weblogs

There are different types of weblogs, or blogs, as they are known. They can be written by any individual who wants to share their ideas, knowledge or experiences online. The two most common types of blog are described as social media and include the microblogs Twitter and Facebook, where each entry is referred to as a 'post'. You can 'add' or 'follow' users or groups so you receive information on your newsfeed on a regular basis to see and share up-to-date information. This is another good way of keeping up to date, but you must not post anything which could bring your registration into question (NMC 2015d).

Providing evidence

You are required to maintain accurate and verifiable records of your CPD activities and you should keep these records for three years until your next revalidation cycle is due to begin. Evidence may include emails, audit tools or guidelines you have developed, copies of presentations, notes, course certificates, signed letters, reflective accounts or conference programmes. This is not an exhaustive list (see Chapter 10 on portfolio development for more information).

Using CPD to support revalidation

There are a number of case studies below from practitioners showing how they have used everyday events to support their CPD.

Case study 1

Maria James is a nurse working in community. She attends her team meetings every month and is looking to find opportunities for CPD. She discusses this with her colleagues and decides to consider what she has learned from her meetings and how this has influenced her practice. While reflecting, Maria realizes that she had asked a clinical question about wound dressing choice and received peer support to answer this question. She then applied this learning in practice. This activity is CPD which she can then record as individual and participatory learning for revalidation purposes.

Case study 2

Bobby Eastwood works as a lecturer and spends most of his time educating and supporting nursing and midwifery students. During a group session he is asked a challenging question about an element of practice he was teaching. This leads to him considering the evidence from the literature and spending a few hours researching the answer. He then shares this with his students and colleagues. This activity is CPD which Bobby could then include in his portfolio as individual and participatory learning as part of his revalidation evidence.

Case study 3

Joanna Barns is an independent midwife who works on her own most of the time. When thinking about meeting the NMC's CPD requirements, Joanna starts to consider how she can interact with others to support her participatory learning. This is the area causing Joanna most anxiety as a sole practitioner. Joanna decides to make a plan of her CPD opportunities – she identifies a number of opportunities where she attends professional seminars and plans to build up her professional network. She also has contact with other independent midwives and obstetricians through her work and decides to discuss with them how they can support each other with CPD and revalidation. Joanna recognizes that her participatory learning may be in an online environment, rather than face-to-face.

Example completed continuing professional development (CPD) record

You should provide information about each learning activity using the most up-to-date headings as required by the NMC (NMC 2015e). See Table 4.5 for an example of a record of a CPD activity. Always check the NMC website for the most up-to-date information and templates, complete a record for every CPD activity you undertake, and keep this record either electronically or in paper format. You must also ensure anonymity at all times by not naming other staff or service users, whether they are alive or deceased (NMC 2015e).

Table 4.5 Example of completed CPD record

Date the CPD was undertaken	30/05/2016
Method of CPD – e.g. online learning, study day.	Senior Charge Nurse Forum Topic – 'Update on Standards for Older People and Preparing for Inspections'. Face-to-face learning event with discussion and questions from the senior nursing group.
A brief description of the key points of the topic, how it relates to your scope of practice, including any learning and how you have applied this.	From the afternoon session the topic which was of most relevance to my clinical practice was 'A Day in the Life of a Healthcare Inspector'.

Key points

- Discussion on the origins and purpose of inspectorate visits.
- Areas of enquiry from inspectors.
- Preparing your staff for visits – providing evidence and ensuring practice reflects safe and effective care.

Scope

As a charge nurse it is my responsibility to ensure my area meets the standard required by the inspectorate.

Learning

This activity gave me increased insight into the key priorities for inspectors and suggestions as to how to prepare more robustly for future inspections. This included how to link clinical practice and activity into building evidence and demonstrating good practice within my clinical area.

Application

I have discussed the learning from this event with my team to raise awareness of the key issues. We have reviewed the inspection-based assessment criteria for our clinical area and identified areas of good practice and where focus is needed.

(Continued)

Table 4.5 (Continued)

Links to the part(s) of the Code.	Practise Effectively and Preserve Safety.
Number of hours. (Describing whether these are individual or participatory learning.)	Two hours total including two hours participatory.
CPD activity evidence.	Notes I took from the session.

Summary

This chapter has described different ways you can evidence CPD for the purposes of revalidation. It has given you ideas and examples to help you identify suitable CPD activities for your ongoing professional development.

To meet the NMC revalidation requirements of 35 hours of CPD (including 20 hours of participatory learning), you will need to select the items within your portfolio which best reflect your scope of practice and meet the minimum requirements. You must be prepared to discuss your CPD activities, as well as the other revalidation requirements, with your confirmer.

In the next chapter we will consider another element of revalidation – practice-related feedback.

Key points

- CPD can take place formally or informally. Take every opportunity you can to learn.
- CPD must be related to your scope of practice and should be used to develop your practice.
- CPD should incorporate a variety of activities and link to the Code (NMC 2015a).
- Once you have undertaken any CPD record this in a log as soon as possible.

5 Practice-related feedback

This chapter will define what practice-related feedback is and what this means for you. It will also explore the value of feedback and the use of different models when giving feedback to others.

Feedback is important because it encourages reflection on many areas, including your practice, an event, or your own behaviour. You are required to obtain five pieces of practice-related feedback over the three years before your registration is due to be renewed. By exploring how to seek feedback, the material in this chapter will be of help as you collect evidence to meet your revalidation requirements.

You can choose to use feedback in many different ways, not only for this purpose. Feedback is an essential way of finding out more about how you undertake your role, and so it will be useful to your practice to reflect on the opinions of others and to have a critical discussion in relation to this feedback. This will then benefit or improve your practice which will result in you becoming a more reflective practitioner and may result in better outcomes for patients or clients. As with all aspects of revalidation, check the NMC website (https://www.nmc.org.uk) for the most up-to-date guidance and templates.

Learning objectives

By the end of this chapter you will be able to:

● Explain how feedback is incorporated into the revalidation process.
● Describe what feedback is and list the different types of feedback.

- Learn skills which you can use when giving or discussing feedback.
- Recognize different models which can be used to structure your feedback.
- Ask for feedback from a colleague or peer.

NMC revalidation requirements

The NMC (2015: 18) states that:

'You must have obtained five pieces of practice-related feedback in the three-year period since your registration was last renewed or you joined the register.'

Always refer to the NMC website for the most up-to-date revalidation guidance.

What is feedback?

Feedback is how we learn about ourselves from our experiences and from other people. It is how we learn from life. Learning about ourselves can be challenging though, depending on how the feedback is given and received (Stone and Heen 2015). Feedback is centred around good communication skills, including effective listening skills, which are covered in more detail in Chapter 7. Feedback can be given in many ways, either informally – e.g. a comment from a colleague (see Case studies 1 and 2 below) or formally – e.g. a written performance review (see Case studies 3 and 4 below).

Informal feedback

Case study 1

Newly qualified nurse Mohammed Akmed has just given Mrs A her medication while undertaking a supervised medication round with his mentor. The mentor has chosen to praise Mohammed on his knowledge of the medications being administered as well as the communication skills he has shown in explaining the medication to Mrs A.

This is informal feedback as it has been given verbally and is not part of Mohammed's more formal competencies.

Following this feedback, Mohammed reflected that even when rushed it was important to take time to give full explanations to patients regarding medication and encourage patient or clients to ask questions.

Case study 2

Midwife Joanne Smith works in the Continuing Education Department and has given a presentation to a class on patient safety. One of her class chooses to tell her how much they enjoyed her session, but that they did not quite understand one of the theories discussed. Following this feedback Joanne decides to review the presentation to make this aspect clearer and re-evaluate after she has run the next course.

Formal feedback

Case study 3

Staff nurse Julie Jones has undertaken a course in order to be able to administer intravenous medication (IVs). As part of this she undertook an exam where she needed to obtain 100 per cent in the calculations section and 50 per cent in the remainder of the paper. The paper was marked by the education team and the questions that Julie answered incorrectly included feedback on how to develop the required knowledge and skills. Following this, the plan would be that Julie could then resit the calculations section and be able to begin her supervised practice in IV medication administration.

Case study 4

Health visitor Johan Melville has been undertaking a leadership course as part of his ongoing professional development. This has involved written feedback from peers on his leadership qualities. With his leadership coach he reviews the information given and formulates an action plan to learn from the feedback and incorporate the impact of this learning into his practice.

Feedback should be recorded as it occurs to allow you to detail the context and other useful pieces of information. There are a few ways feedback can be given, and these include:

- Verbal – this could be in person, via phone or video conference. This could be from relatives, patients or clients, peers, colleagues, university staff or students.
- Written – this can be via email or given to you personally (thank you cards can be used provided these are anonymized). It can also include reports or surveys.
- Audio – this could be a digital recording or podcast (this could be useful where the feedback is from a different geographical location to yours).

As you can see, the way feedback can be given varies, and where you seek it from a variety of sources this will widen the views and experiences from which you can learn.

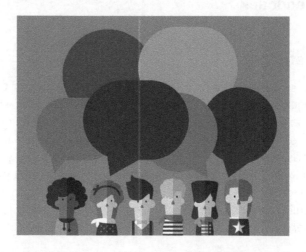

Time Out

Consider the last time you gave feedback to someone. You might want to consider situations within your practice or professional life, and also personal situations – e.g. feedback to a colleague or to a customer service agent.

How was this done? e.g. face-to-face or online.

Was this mainly critical or positive feedback?

How did you feel about giving feedback? Why do you think you felt like this, and did the fact it was critical or positive affect your feelings?

Reflect on your answers and consider how you will address your feelings in the future.

Remember: you may want to log this learning as part of your CPD hours for your revalidation evidence.

When considering feedback in the Time Out box you may have considered a time when you gave feedback within your professional role to students in your area or maybe colleagues who are currently revalidating. In your personal life you may have given feedback regarding something you have bought or a service you have accessed – for example, via an online questionnaire or paper-based questionnaire in a restaurant. In the instances of feedback to a business this will ensure that they improve or continue to provide a service that their customers want to use. This has relevance to healthcare where we want to replicate and continue to do things which are improving practice, and obtain information to improve the areas that perhaps are not being undertaken as well as they could be. In addition, it can provide evidence of your effectiveness as a practitioner and be very encouraging and motivating to your practice. Even if feedback is more critical, this may give you direction in relation to future learning and development as a professional. It is likely that you receive feedback within your practice informally, but perhaps you have not always been aware of it – e.g. your manager praising your input and specific actions that have resulted in a good outcomes (see the case studies of informal and formal feedback earlier). Review the cases below, and consider if they are appropriate to be used as evidence of feedback for revalidation purposes.

Case study 1

Charge nurse Jonathan James works in an acute mental health unit where he was caring for a young girl with a complex mental health condition. Once she had been discharged the family sent a thank you card to the ward. Jonathan decides to photocopy this and use this as feedback.

Case study 2

Midwife Lorraine Wright asks her mentor for feedback in relation to her being responsible for undertaking a pregnant lady's first 'booking in' appointment. The mentor details the elements that were undertaken well and gives some areas of constructive feedback to allow the newly qualified midwife to focus on her continued development.

Case study 3

Staff nurse Lana Millar works in a care home. They have recently received an inspection regarding the care home's performance. Lana decides to use the report as a basis for looking at areas of development and good practice to inform her own development and also share with her colleagues.

What did you think? Case study 1 can be used for feedback, but there is no need to photocopy the card – you are only required to keep a note of any feedback you receive. If Jonathan did want to photocopy this he would need to anonymize it and check with his manager that he can use it as it belongs to the ward. What he could do is reflect on it in a wider context – e.g. acknowledge that positive generic feedback was given, but look to map this to his delivery of care and what he has learned as a result of this. Case studies 2 and 3 are examples that are suitable and may be useful when considering the options within your own practice.

Note that feedback can be for teams as well as individual, but ensure that all the information is freely available and not contraindicating any data protection regulations. Where you wish to use your employer's information you will be required to ask for consent. All information must be anonymized and non-identifiable. Where you involve patients or clients, they should also be informed of your intentions to use the information and told that it will be totally confidential and non-identifiable (NMC 2015e).

How does this link to revalidation?

Always check the NMC website for the most up-to-date information, as this may change. Currently the NMC have a recommended template you can use which allows you to record feedback in relation to:

- The source: this is where the feedback comes from.
- Type of feedback: this is how the feedback was received (see above).
- Content of feedback: what was the feedback about and how is this related to or has it affected your practice?

You can chose to use this template or create one of your own, as long as you capture the NMC revalidation requirements which are that you have obtained at least five pieces of practice-related feedback over the three years prior to you re-registering (NMC 2015e).

When considering what feedback to use, remember it needs to be relevant to your practice. And, as well as ensuring you have the minimum number required, this can also be used to formulate any of your five reflections required for revalidation purposes. You will usually receive feedback as part of your annual appraisal, which means you should have received at least three pieces of feedback during each revalidation cycle – this makes things a bit easier as feedback will automatically be incorporated into your review. This feedback should allow both parties an opportunity to give and receive feedback from each other.

It is useful to use a variety of sources for feedback, which are discussed next.

Who can give you feedback?

Time Out

Who do you think could give you feedback, and why? Consider what kind of feedback you receive on a day-to-day basis – for example, from students, service users, managers or colleagues.

Other ways of obtaining feedback include the use of reports or audits which are within the public domain (i.e. not confidential), or complaints; but again, remember to ask permission to use these and remove any personal information. These reports and documents may give feedback about your unit or ward, the team that you are part of, or the larger organization. The most important part of this is to make the feedback meaningful and detail how you will use the feedback to improve your practice. Utilizing a variety of sources and individuals can provide a range of feedback which is most beneficial to the development of your practice.

Pause for Thought

Why do you think some people do not like to give or receive feedback?

Consider a time when you didn't seek feedback or didn't give feedback and reflect on why this might have been the case.

In thinking about this you may have detailed the following:

- Fear – of the unknown or the process. Also fear of critical feedback which may worry the individual in relation to their professional reputation.
- Stress – being overloaded and not feeling able to hear feedback.
- Lack of confidence – regarding the skills for the process or individual performance.

- Not being familiar with feedback – it may not have occurred to you to give, or recognize, when you are receiving feedback.
- Previous bad experience with the process of feedback, which may be helpful to explore.
- Time to undertake the process.
- Low self-esteem – a belief that you do not have positive experiences or events to get feedback on.

When considering the reasons you don't like to receive feedback, you may have reflected on the reasons why this is the case, and identified some learning needs. This is an opportunity for you to recognize the real benefits of receiving feedback in relation to developing your practice.

If you are unsure how to give feedback in a way that does not cause conflict or offence, using one of the models described next can help to address these concerns.

Models of feedback

As a registered nurse or midwife there is an expectation that, as a professional, you will be able to give and receive feedback. Where this skill is new to you, or you want to improve how you give feedback, you may wish to use a model. Some models are detailed below as examples, but you may wish to use another, or be skilled in this already.

Time Out

Ask a peer or colleague how they give feedback and whether they utilize a model or not. If they use a model, ask them which one; try it out with a colleague you trust, and see how it feels for you.

By practising giving feedback in an informal setting first gives you an idea of how this will feel when you have to do this in practice.

Feedback sandwich

This is where you start and end with a positive with the middle part being constructive or more critical feedback (Daniels 2009).

The idea behind this is that it is, overall, a positive experience with focused learning. The first part is finding something related, close in time, and significant that the individual did well, and starting with this. Hopefully, the individual will feel supported and receptive when you then present constructive facts in a non-judgemental, firm manner. End with a positive aspect so that this redresses any negative emotions the constructive feedback may have evoked in the individual. Where possible, do not wait until the next issue arises to follow up the actions required (see example in Box 5.1).

Box 5.1: Example using the sandwich model

Staff nurse Elspeth Biggs has drafted some information for patients on protected mealtimes within her clinical setting. The charge nurse uses a 'feedback sandwich' to give her feedback on her leaflet.

Charge nurse:

'Elspeth, that was an excellent idea to draft an information leaflet for patients; it is something that is needed for patients.' (*Positive*)

'There are a couple of amendments I would like to suggest which are that the hospital would like all communications to look similar, with their logo and layout.' (*Constructive*)

'However, after these amendments, I hope we will be able to get it printed. And I am sure many patients will benefit from this – thanks for undertaking this project.' (*Positive*)

The example above showed that the charge nurse gave constructive advice to make the leaflet better, but praised the actions and efforts that Elspeth had put in. Any negative emotions felt were counteracted by the positive praise at the end, with the hope that this will result in the changes being made and a good outcome for patients – hence the name, 'Sandwich Model'.

As with other models, it is important to carefully plan what you are going to say and structure it accordingly. This will ensure that you cover the points that you wish to make, and that you are leading and controlling the conversation. A potential issue with this model is where it is used every time the person is then 'ready' for the critical or constructive feedback, and therefore may consciously or unconsciously blank out the positive feedback. Where appropriate, backing this up with written feedback may assist; or use another model, such as *Pendleton's rules*, which is discussed next as an alternative.

Pendleton's rules

Pendleton's rules (Pendleton et al. 1984) are seen as a framework to give balanced feedback so that both positive and critical aspects are explored, and the person giving feedback is referred to as an 'observer'.

They described the following process:

1   Check firstly that the person is ready and wants feedback. This will then clarify the process.
2   Ask for the person's perspective on what has gone well, and any other comments or background to the topic or event that is being discussed.
3   The observer details what has gone well.
4   The person states what could have been done better or differently. This then may include suggestions for change, or what could be improved.
5   The observer states how it could be improved, which may be options for change.
6   An action plan for improvement is agreed and formulated.

Example using Pendleton's rules

Janice Neeson is a mental health nurse working in the clinical governance department for a health and social care locality. Her manager, Kathy Rodgers, has reviewed a new policy she has drafted and, using Pendleton's rules, gives feedback, as shown below.

Kathy Rodgers (KR): Hi Janice, I see you have completed the draft policy, would it be possible to give you some feedback on this when you are available?

Janice Neeson (JN): Hi. That is great. I was hoping you would have had a chance to look at it and am free now if you want.

KR: *Great. Firstly, this was your first time drafting a policy, so how do you feel it went given it had a large number of stakeholders involved?*

JN: *The actual policy draft was fairly straightforward as I followed the examples you gave me and the organizational template.*

KR: *I would agree regarding the format – it has very much followed the guidelines which is what was required. I think maybe a few words could be changed slightly, and I have highlighted these in the document. Is there anything you thought could have been done better?*

JN: *I found getting staff to engage with the process of developing the policy and getting feedback on this very challenging. They would arrange to meet me and then cancel, which was frustrating.*

KR: *That does sound challenging and indeed frustrating. It really is important to get their views so it is done in collaboration. Do you think taking the draft to the team meetings may be something that would be an option going forward?*

JN: *That sounds a good approach. I will contact the areas and set up meetings next week.*

This model can provide a useful framework and you may wish to try it out on a friend to see how it feels first before you try it in practice. Walsh (2005) was critical of this model, citing that this is not how things occur in 'real life', and that it can be problematic, especially when dealing with junior staff. However, using a model you are happy with is important, and there are others available by searching the internet or asking colleagues.

As well as using a model to structure your feedback you also need to consider that the feedback you give is good quality. There is an acronym you can use to help remember this: **BOOST**, as explained in Table 5.1, which helps you consider how to give or prepare the feedback (Clayton 2012).

Whatever model you decide (or do not decide) to use there are some key principles which promote good feedback. When considering feedback in the context of formal education, for example, if you are a lecturer or work in education role and give feedback to students, you may find the Higher Education Academy's (HEA) seven principles of good feedback practice helpful. These are shown in Table 5.2.

Table 5.1 BOOST model (Clayton 2012)

Balanced	Include both good and bad points.
Observed	Only give examples of what you have observed them doing, rather than your own opinion or hearsay.
Objective or owned	Be factual – keep any emotions to one side.
Specific	Always use specific examples to illustrate a comment and exactly how or why was this done well or badly.
Timely	Always give the feedback as close to the event as possible to ensure accuracy and effectiveness.

Table 5.2 Key principles for successful feedback (Juwah et al. 2004)

Principle	Additional information
1. The process facilitates the development of self-assessment in learning.	This is related to reflective practice and Chapter 6 will cover this in further detail.
2. Encourages teacher and peer dialogue around learning.	Talking about learning before feedback can be utilized for your own development needs.
3. Helps clarify what good performance is (goals, criteria and standards expected).	This has the benefits of being more specific and measurable leading to more chance of improvement and success.
4. Provides opportunities to close the gap between current and desired performance.	By discussing the actual performance in real time, and the desired outcome, allows development of an action plan or specifying what is required. This would work best with timescales identified and any resources that will be required detailed too.
5. Delivers high-quality information to students about their learning.	This requires the observer or coach to do preparation to ensure the information given is clear, defined and gives enough detail for change to be understood and planned by the individual. Where you are giving or receiving feedback, try to ensure it is specific and clear.
6. Encourages positive motivational beliefs and self-esteem.	To ensure this is possible, feedback needs to make the individual feel valued and positive despite an element where development or change of behaviour is required. See models of giving feedback.
7. Provides information to teachers that can be used to help shape the teaching.	This could be interpreted as two-way communication and feedback so both parties benefit.

In addition to these there are also some other aspects that can make the experience more meaningful. These are applicable to both formal and informal feedback and include:

- Time. Give feedback when asked (e.g. for revalidation purposes) or, if it is in relation to an event, as soon as possible after the event – e.g. a colleague asking how you think her presentation went after a conference the next day, rather than waiting. Ensure you have enough time to fully discuss the event and have a critical discussion.
- Seeking out opportunities for feedback. Where feedback is part of a formal event – e.g. appraisal – this tends to occur as it is part of the process. However, opportunities for receiving feedback from others could involve approaching them informally.
- Choose a venue that is private and confidential (see also Chapter 7) if you are giving difficult and/or more formal feedback.
- Overall, try and focus on the positive and suggest development needs in a supportive, positive manner.
- The content of the feedback needs to be about the event or the opinion sought; do not bring up previous concerns or mistakes. Where possible, give specific examples and focus on behaviours, not personality traits. Do not be afraid to use 'I' to give examples and detail your experience of the event. Keep the messages clear and do not overload the feedback with multiple different events or subjects.
- Where the feedback is critical or of a more constructive nature try to suggest alternative ways to approach the issue so they have something to work on.
- Remember the feedback is for that individual and therefore be aware and sensitive to verbal and non-verbal cues as to how the message is being received. Use communication techniques such as good verbal and non-verbal skills, as well as development of mutual respect and trust. Watch out for your verbal and non-verbal communication not matching – e.g. giving praise, but your body language suggesting barriers and defensiveness (see also Chapter 7).
- Engage and develop your reflective skills as this will help you as a registrant and if you take on the role of reflective discussion partner (see Chapters 6 and 7).

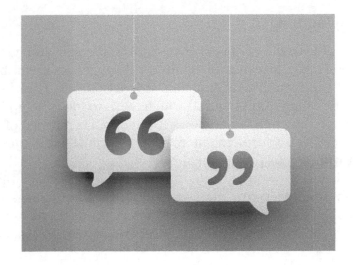

Receiving feedback

Feedback should be part of your day-to-day practice; however, because of the revalidation process you may become more aware of how feedback is given and received within your area. Part of this process will be you being prepared to receive feedback – and sometimes hearing even positive feedback can feel uncomfortable!

The following tips may help when you are preparing to receive feedback:

- Professionalism – always keep within professional boundaries.
- Listen to the feedback carefully and try not to get emotional. Ask for it to be repeated or clarified if necessary. Try not to immediately prepare a 'defence' or counterargument.
- If it is constructive or critical then consider the comments carefully and ask for clarification, or an example, if it is not clear what they are alluding to. Try to breathe deeply and pause to take in the information, especially if you are naturally a reflective individual.
- Try not to dismiss the information, but accept it positively. Asking them for ways to improve or change can be helpful here.
- Remember to build mutual trust and respect.
- Where the feedback is detailed or complex, ask for this to be in written format.

Links to learning

In the adult learning chapter (Chapter 3) Kolb's learning cycle was discussed (1984). This has relevance to feedback as it can be seen as part of experiential learning. Kolb's model showed a link between learning by doing (experiential) which leads to ideas being formed and reshaped through experiences. This supports the idea of you as a nurse or midwife becoming more reflective and encourages development within your professional role. Where feedback is linked to an experience or event with clear learning outcomes then the feedback can be utilized to complement the overall outcomes of that programme – e.g. feedback on preparing a syringe driver could also be part of the supervised practice involved in being competent at this skill.

Summary

This chapter has explored what feedback is and the different types you can utilize for your revalidation evidence. The models described can be used to structure the way you give feedback and allow you to understand how feedback may be given to you. Practising giving and receiving both positive and more critical or constructive feedback will enhance and improve your skills in relation to this, and you can share these tips with your colleagues. The next chapter explores reflection, which can also be used to enhance the way you learn from feedback.

Key points

- Feedback can be given either formally or informally.
- Using a model to give feedback can help you structure this more carefully, particularly when you are giving more constructive feedback.
- Always take time to make a note of any feedback you receive and consider how you can use this to improve your practice.

CHAPTER

6 Reflection

Reflection in and on practice is fundamental to good care provision within nursing and midwifery practice. This chapter will seek to demystify what is meant by reflection and reflective practice, and provide examples of models and tools. Having a basic understanding of reflection is important for revalidation as you have to complete five written reflective accounts and have a reflective discussion with another registrant (this is covered in more detail in Chapter 7). However, it is acknowledged that for some individuals engaging in reflection may be new, and this chapter contains theory to set the scene, and examples to 'bring it to life'.

Learning objectives

By the end of the chapter you will be able to:

● Define the terms 'reflection' and 'reflective practice'.
● Describe different types of reflective models that can be utilized.
● Apply a model to undertake a reflective account that can be used to provide evidence for revalidation.

Current NMC revalidation requirements

The NMC (2015: 20) states that:

You must have prepared five written reflective accounts in the three-year period since your registration was last renewed or you joined the register. Each reflective account must be recorded on the approved form and must refer to:

an instance of your CPD and/or a piece of practice-related feedback you have received and/or an event or experience in your own professional practice and how this relates to the Code.

Always refer to the NMC website for the most up-to-date revalidation guidance.

What is reflection?

The term reflection is derived from the Latin term 'reflectere' – meaning 'to bend back'. Reflection involves reviewing experience from practice so that it can be described, analysed and evaluated. Reflection is a process of making sense of experience in order to move on and do better as a practitioner (Bulman et al. 2012), thus it can inform and change future practice (Bulman and Schutz 2008). Utilizing reflection within health and social care has key benefits for our patients, service users and the profession. Reflection can be utilized before, during and after an event, all of which can allow improvements to be made through learning. In some aspects of nursing this has been a key aspect of practice for a long time – e.g. mental health and learning disability nursing where reflection both as an individual, with other professionals and with service users may be practised. Reflection could also be described as:

- Thinking about.
- Pondering on.
- Asking yourself questions about.
- Discussing with yourself.
- Trying to work something out or making sense of things.
- Learning from experience.
- Helping you plan your actions in the future.

Reflection can also foster mindfulness which is about being engaged fully to allow this awareness to be utilized in our daily lives. Siegel (2007) states that mindfulness helps us awaken, and by reflection on the mind we are enabled to make choices and allow change to be embraced.

Why formal reflection?

The revalidation process has made reflection mandatory and there-fore it needs to become an aspect of your practice. However, reflection has always been something that healthcare professionals should have engaged with. Indeed, it has become widely regarded as important as it provides a way of learning from practice (Bowman and Addyman 2014). It was first described by Dewey (1933), followed by Schön (1983), who devised the concept of the 'reflective practitioner'. It is important to note that reflection can and should be on both positive and negative experiences and, for revalidation purposes, also relate to aspects of your practice in relation to the Code (NMC 2015a). Choosing events that highlight both areas for development and those where things have gone well provides valuable learning (Stonehouse 2011). It is also important to note that reflection can occur not just on a critical incident, but on more naturalistic experiences, and that critical incident analysis is not the same as reflection.

The Nursing & Midwifery Council has stated that:

'The Code will be central in the revalidation process as a focus for professional reflection. This will give the Code significance in your professional life, and raise its status and importance for employers (NMC 2015e).'

Within the Code (NMC 2015a: 8) reflection is further detailed in the following parts:

You reflect and act on any feedback you receive to improve your practice.

9.1 provide honest, accurate and constructive feedback to colleagues.

9.2 gather and reflect on feedback from a variety of sources, using it to improve your practice and performance.

24.2 use all complaints as a form of feedback and an opportunity for reflection and learning to improve practice.

It is therefore essential that reflection becomes an integral part of your practice.

Firstly, do not worry that you will not have examples that will work for reflection as it is an area that can cover many aspects of your practice. Consider the following list of opportunities where reflection can occur, and start by choosing one which you feel comfortable with within your current role.

Box 6.1: Opportunities which can be used to reflect

- Hand-over times or team meetings.
- Teaching sessions – structured or unstructured, clinical or non-clinical.
- Working with staff members who have different skills to you – this may be staff of another grade and may be individuals with different examples of skills or activities that you do not possess.
- Reflection in the car – either alone or with a colleague following a clinical visit in the community.
- Reading a journal or article – this may be as an individual or a part of a journal club.
- Participating in discussion at a journal club or as an agenda item at a team meeting (this can be linked to areas of specific interest and or professional roles – e.g. 'link' nurse roles).
- Networking meetings.
- Conferences – this can be linked to the main plenary sessions or workshops where they can be more interactive.
- Case conferences – these can be multiprofessional or multi-agency and may be internal – e.g. within a ward environment, or external – e.g. a children's panel.
- Mentoring or preceptorship discussions.
- Maintaining a professional portfolio.
- Clinical risk assessments.
- Clinical audits.
- Ward or team meetings.
- Discussion and analysis regarding critical incidents or near misses within practice.

As you read these, reflect upon which opportunities you personally resolve to engage in and those which you can encourage your mentor and other colleagues to engage in. Write this up in your portfolio and review your progress at regular intervals (see also Chapter 10).

Time Out

What journals do you read at work? Make a list of those that are general – e.g. *Nursing Standard*, *Nursing Times*, *British Journal of Nursing*, or those that are specific to your area of practice – e.g. *International Journal of Older People Nursing*, *Orthopaedic Nursing Journal* etc.

How could you use these to reflect on your practice either as an individual, a group, or a journal club?

You may want to consider logging these hours as either individual or participatory CPD hours for revalidation.

Lifelong learning is an essential part of being a professional, and continuing to develop throughout your career has clear benefits (see also Chapter 3 and 4). Reflection feeds into this as it is a type of deeper thinking designed to help us gain a better understanding of ourselves, our values, knowledge and skills. It allows us to learn from our experiences and supports personal growth which enables us to adapt and respond to new challenges. It is therefore important to develop your practice through the process of reflection.

Reflection can be likened to looking in a mirror; however, Fowler (2014) urges practitioners to view reflection as something that takes us one step further than a mirror, which can often be only a swift superficial glance. Fowler suggests instead using the analogy of a microscope, where we take a closer look to allow deeper evaluation and learning from practice. Specific skills will help you in the reflective process, and these include self-awareness and being able to utilize skills of analysis. Both will be discussed later in the chapter.

Reflection is used in a variety of contexts. For instance, 'action learning' utilizes reflection by building 'on the relationship between reflection and action' (McGill and Brockbank 2004) and usually involves being a member of an action learning set. Clinical supervision also utilizes reflection with the focus on clinically analysing situations to promote development. It is usually between two individuals and is often seen by organizations as a way to promote personal and professional development in their staff (Jasper 2006). (Also see Chapter 8.)

You may be coming to this chapter having gained some level of skill in reflective practice, have some knowledge of reflection, or already be aware that your knowledge and skills could improve in relation to reflective practice. Using the flow diagram in Figure 6.1 you can determine how to use this chapter and plan your further development in this area.

Pause for Thought

Think about where you are currently and whether you reflect.

How do you reflect on your practice? Do you do this in the car on the way home or through discussion with colleagues or family?

How formal is it – do you write anything down? What feels best for you and why?

Reflection is a powerful tool to enable learning from our experiences and has been shown to provide valuable professional development for a range of healthcare practitioners, not just nursing (Oelofsen 2012). Whether reflection is carried out formally or informally it is of great importance within the revalidation process, enabling you to learn and improve your practice.

What elements are involved in reflection?

In order to develop as a reflective practitioner, the following elements are key:

- Emotional intelligence.
- Self-awareness.
- Critical analysis.

Each element will now be explored, and you are encouraged to think about the experience you can gain and development opportunities that can be undertaken to improve in these areas.

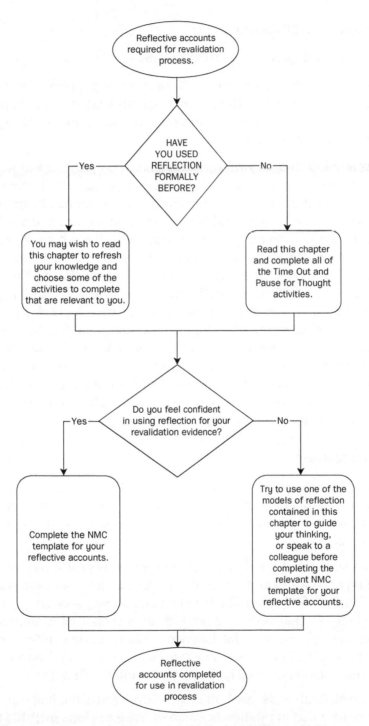

Figure 6.1 Exploring your skills in relation to reflective practice

Emotional intelligence

Emotional intelligence can be defined as:

'The ability to recognize one's own and other people's emotions to discriminate between different feelings and label them appropriately, and to use emotional information to guide thinking and behaviour' (Coleman 2008).

Within nursing and midwifery, caring and compassion are key elements of your practice, and therefore emotional intelligence is an important attribute to have when caring for patients, clients or service users. As nursing and midwifery are both an art and a science, with frequent learning experienced while working within the clinical environment (experiential learning), this can indeed be improved by having emotional intelligence. However, Goleman (1996) states that this can sometimes get in the way of logical understanding and judgements, and therefore our actions can get clouded. Practising reflection will encourage development of emotional intelligence, and learning to control emotions can promote a better learning experience. Even if you are new to the process of formal reflection it is likely that you have reflected in an informal way within your practice as a nurse or midwife, and this may have included reflecting on your feelings about an element of your practice.

Self-awareness

Self-awareness is an essential part of reflection and learning. Atkins and Shutz (2013) describe being self-aware as: 'to be conscious of one's character, including beliefs, values, qualities, strengths and limitations'.

What is clear is that emotional intelligence requires self-awareness and an ability to be warm and empathetic to develop interpersonal relationships (Hurley 2008). A bit like the chicken and egg scenario, Grainger (2010) believes that reflective practice also assists in facilitating the development of emotional intelligence. Within practice, self-awareness and participation in reflective practice have been recognized as vital in supporting person-centred care (Devenny and Duffy 2013).

It can be difficult to assess how self-aware we are, but it is suggested you consider this in relation to some of the questions in Table 6.1.

Table 6.1 Assessing how self-aware you think you are

Tick the appropriate column for you	Unsure or not undertaken recently	Fairly recently	Very recently	This is part of my regular practice
When was the last time you considered how you came across to colleagues (in other words, how did your behaviour affect others?)				
When was the last time you asked others about how you are perceived?				

If you have a critical friend or mentor who you trust, perhaps ask them their opinion and compare that with your views. You could also ask a close friend or family member as this will impact on both your personal and professional life. You may wish to log this feedback as part of your revalidation evidence.

Even if you are self-aware there is probably room for improvement. Self-awareness can be linked to your values (what is important to you) and motivations (what drives you). Siegel (2007) considers this further and believes that mindful awareness involves reflection on emerging events. This may be something you wish to explore further and practise.

Time Out

Write down what you think your values and motivations are?

Consider how this impacts on your practice and the way you form relationships within the workplace.

How do you think you could become more self-aware? Does this link into aspects of mindfulness for you?

Who do you think could help you to become more self-aware?

Possible answers may include:

- Spending time considering what your values and motivations are. Have they changed? If you are comfortable discussing this with a friend, colleague or critical friend it may help plan possible developments for you.
- Being brave and asking how self-aware your colleagues at work perceive you to be. This should be undertaken by utilizing those you trust, seeking an honest opinion – perhaps using a 'critical friend', a mentor, or previous mentor within your workplace (see Chapter 8). In addition, family members or friends outside work may be interesting to compare and contrast answers. Furthermore, be aware you may get different answers based on the individual, the situation, and whether the person sees you in work or in your personal life outside of work, as we all tend to operate differently in work and home environments.
- Self-analysis of verbal and non-verbal feedback from patients, colleagues or service users who have commented on your practice.

Pause for Thought

Think of someone you consider self-aware.

What advantages do you see for this individual both for themselves and others?

Would you consider them as a role model?

Johari's window

The Johari window was created by two American psychologists, Joseph Luft (1916–2014) and Harrington Ingham (1914–95) in 1955. It is a simplistic diagram with four quadrants which assist in understanding and developing self-awareness, improving interpersonal relationships and communication and development of self (and others). The four quadrants contain regions that include: 1. Open/free area, 2. Blind area, 3. Hidden area and 4. Unknown areas (see Figure 6.2).

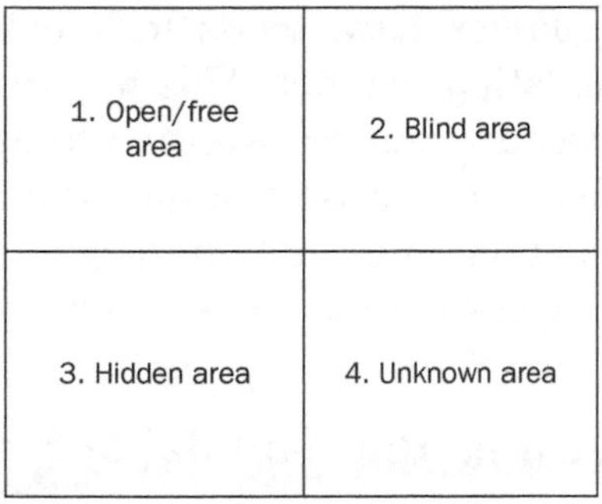

1. Open/free area	2. Blind area
3. Hidden area	4. Unknown area

Figure 6.2 Johari's window

Despite the figure showing all of the quadrants as the same size, they can be altered to represent proportions of knowledge about a group and/or individuals.

Quadrant 1: Open/free area

This is information which is known by both the person (self) and others, group or team.

The biggest advantage to having this area is that there are no hidden aspects. Information here can be used to promote good relationships based on trust, understanding and good communication. Conversely, aspects within this quadrant can also reduce or diminish misinterpretation and feelings of being threatened, or confusion and conflict.

Example: Senior nurse, Bridget Weinburg, has experience in dealing with patients with a diagnosis of Cancer of an Unknown Primary (CUP), which often includes managing complex cases. Both the senior nurse and other members of the clinical team have confidence and trust in the other nurses being assigned a patient with this diagnosis.

Quadrant 2: Blind self/blind spot or blind area

This is what is known about a person by others, but is unknown by the person. Although this may sound quite intimidating it can be overcome by becoming more self-aware, which includes seeking feedback from others.

Example: Midwife, James Law, tends to speak to new members of staff in an intimidating manner. This has resulted in new team members feeling insecure and not wanting to ask questions. When James sought feedback, this aspect of his practice was highlighted in a supportive way and it allowed him to change some of the communication skills he was exhibiting in relation to this.

Quadrant 3: Known as the 'façade' or hidden area

This is what is known to ourselves, but is not disclosed to others; thus, they are unaware of this hidden aspect. Often this area is one where sensitivity is required due to feelings, fear and insecurities. In some instances they can include aspects not related to work, and therefore disclosure is not deemed appropriate from the individual's perspective. However, where this is work related, it is much better to be voiced as it leads to better teamworking, trust and communication.

Example: Student nurse, Elizabeth Nowak, has previously been involved in a car accident. On placement in Accident and Emergency a patient is admitted with an injury due to a car accident. Staff are aware Elizabeth is behaving differently, but only understand the situation when she chooses to disclose this. The result is that other staff offer her support and help her seek strategies to cope with this in the future.

Quadrant 4: Unknown area or unknown self

This is information unknown to both the individual and other members of the group or team. Caution is to be exercised in this region as it may include traumatic aspects from past events which are unresolved. However, it can also be very powerful in development where allowing a safe environment to develop and experiment promotes a way of 'trying out' new skills which can increase motivation and interest in job satisfaction.

Example: Staff nurse, Brian Hemsly, works in a general medical ward, but has to escort a patient for dialysis, an area that they have not previously worked in. He finds the complexities and technical aspect of dialysis to be of great interest, and wishes to learn more. He had not previously been aware of his interest in this aspect of care, and it has been motivating to have the opportunity to 'try this out'.

Where disclosure stems from previous trauma, it should be stressed that this would not be expected to be dealt with in the workplace, but would require professional counselling due to the distress this could cause to the individual (McGill and Brockbank 2004).

Altering the quadrant areas

This can be achieved in different ways, dependent on the area being explored.

The open area can be developed through a process of sharing information about yourself. The blind area can be reduced by feedback (both asking and receiving). The hidden area often involves disclosure which the individual feels comfortable in sharing. Finally, the unknown area can be altered through self-discovery or development which may include you accessing coaching and mentoring to help you explore this aspect.

Time Out

Use Johari's model to look at what you share with your team or self-disclosure. What do you think you could do to improve aspects for you as an individual? Do you have a team development day or activity that could involve utilizing this model within the team?

Remember that, even if this is challenging, undertaking this activity can help to reduce conflict, improve communication, and encourage self and team growth, leading to better teamwork and improved practice.

Critical analysis

Atkins (cited in Burns and Bulman 2000) highlights that terms such as critical reflection, critical thinking, critical awareness and critical analysis are, on occasions, used interchangeably, which may compound confusion and anxiety. In relation to reflection it was acknowledged that during the critical analysis stage of a reflective cycle or process (see later) critical thinking is a key element in identifying and exploring alternative approaches.

Primarily, this involves assessing all possible actions or interventions and being able to make reasoned and rational choices following this (Jasper 2013). Again, this can be a skill which can be improved with practice, and when starting, using a friend or colleague with experience may be of benefit. As mentioned previously, using reflection in this way is not the same as critical incident analysis.

Types of models: Why use a model?

Reflective models are useful for the novice reflector, but it is important that the person undertaking the reflection understands the point of reflection and does not over describe the event, but engages in a level of analysis to understand and learn from their experience. The idea of using a model of reflection is to help the formalization of the process and give structure to thoughts and feelings (Stonehouse 2011; Fowler 2014). Indeed, Timmins and Duffy (2011) feel that without this, experiences turn into lists or descriptions rather than evidence of professional competence.

The most important aspect of choosing a model is one which appeals to you and can assist in the description and analysis of an event to show reflection and learning. It may be that a simplistic model is utilized initially, and when you become comfortable another model may be adopted. Jasper (2013) believes that the majority of frameworks and models comprise six stages, including:

Stage One: Selecting a critical incident to reflect on.
Stage Two: Observing and describing the experience.
Stage Three: Analysing the experience.
Stage Four: Interpreting the experience.
Stage Five: Exploring alternatives.
Stage Six: Framing action.

However, Timmins and Duffy (2011) point out that in relation to choosing a model, incorporating a critical element is of use.

They explain that this does not equate with being negative, but goes beyond the boundaries of just personal introspection. This can then lead to key benefits in relation to considering a wider viewpoint that may include the opinions of others, practice in general, policy, knowledge and procedures which lead to action within the practice environment (Timmins and Duffy 2011).

Types of reflection

There are two types of reflection you may have come across already. These are described by Schön as reflection *on* action and reflection *in* action (Schön 1983).

Reflection on action

The first one is reflection 'on action', described by Schön in 1983. This refers to looking back and reflecting on an event that has already taken place. It is likely you will have done this informally as this usually occurs following a significant event at work – e.g. a particularly difficult event with a patient, such as a cardiac arrest, or a relative who is unhappy with the care of their loved one. Questions you may have asked yourself, or as part of your team in these situations, might include:

- What were the things that were going on before the event?
- How did I/the team respond to the event?
- What did we do well, and what could be improved?
- Does anything need to change following this event? What could be done better for patients/relatives/others? Were there any practical aspects which would be changed? These may be small aspects of care, and not necessarily incidents requiring formal action.

Although reflection can be done as an individual, a team approach can be beneficial in covering multiple aspects of practice resulting in innovative ways to improve practice.

Reflection in action

Reflection 'in action' is where reflection occurs during an event, and usually only involves the individual who is reflecting. Schön (1983) advises that this has limitations which need to be acknowledged, and that for success reflection in action needs to be mastered with experience. To give an example, a practitioner performing a complex clinical skill for the first time would find reflecting 'in action' challenging as they may require all their concentration to successfully undertake the activity. However, when skilled, this can be undertaken allowing other aspects such as environment, the patient's response, verbal and non-verbal feedback, and so on, to be considered, thus allowing reflection on the skill while performing the skill. Fowler (2014) gives an example where he claims reflection in action is like driving a car: you are performing a skill which becomes routine with practice, but while undertaking this you are monitoring other road users, road conditions, weather etc., and in doing so at times modify and adjust your own driving to ensure safety and comfort. Fowler concludes by advising that reflection in action is both difficult and requires a degree of honesty and self-awareness.

We will now briefly consider different models of reflection you may find useful, before finally looking at pitfalls to avoid, and then key points to note when logging your reflections.

Gibbs' reflective cycle

This approach has similarities to that of Kolb's learning cycle (1984) (see Chapter 3), and can be utilized to put reflections into a written format, and used as evidence of learning. In order to make the reflection meaningful it requires more than a quick superficial 'tick in the box'. This is improved and enriched by honesty, and if you feel a resistance when exploring it is useful to ask yourself why. Exploring this could unleash fear of disclosing inadequate skills or knowledge, and this needs to be worked through for successful reflection to occur.

Gibbs' (1988) reflective cycle is a popular model for reflection and an adapted version is shown in Figure 6.3. The model includes six stages of reflection and is presented below with a worked example from John Hastie (see Table 6.2), who is a community psychiatric nurse (CPN). He has anonymized the client's name by calling her Mrs A and ensuring he doesn't mention specific details about Mrs A which could identify her.

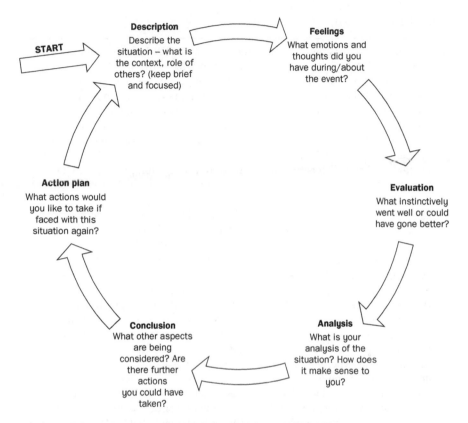

Figure 6.3 Gibbs' reflective cycle (adapted from Gibbs 1988)

Table 6.2 An example of written reflection using Gibbs' reflective cycle

Stage	Example reflection
1. **Description**: In this section, you need to explain what you are reflecting with details to give context, which may include background information. Try to be concise and clear without needless detail.	Mrs A is a lady with schizophrenia. She has been under my caseload for around 18 months. She lives alone and has delusions which are predominantly controlled by medication. When she has acute episodes this can result in hospitalization which causes her more distress. This episode describes me (John) visiting her in hospital as part of a multidisciplinary team meeting to prepare for discharge. When at the meeting Mrs A describes the fact that she feels let down by community services which resulted in her admission.

(Continued)

Table 6.2 (Continued)

2. **Feelings**: Discuss your feelings and thoughts about the experience. Consider questions such as: How did you feel at the time? What did you think at the time? What did you think about the incident afterwards? Ensure a professional tone, whilst being honest.	I feel that as a CPN I am very aware of my responsibilities for Mrs A and what is within my remit. This involves routine appointments to evaluate how medication is controlling Mrs A's symptoms. The criticism of community services came as a surprise, and I am disappointed to hear Mrs A felt like this. I wonder if anything else could have been put in place for her to prevent admission to hospital. While reflecting on the last visit, where things appeared to be fine, I ask myself, 'Did I miss anything?'
3. **Evaluation**: For your evaluation, discuss how well you think things went. Perhaps think about: How did you react to the situation, and how did other people react? What was good and what was bad about the experience? If you are writing about a difficult incident, did you feel that the situation was resolved afterwards? Why/why not? This section is a good place to include the theory and the work of other authors – remember it is important to include references in reflective writing.	As part of the evaluation I looked back on the notes from her appointment. I am reassured to see that I documented the visit, including symptoms, medication management and how Mrs A was feeling. It would appear that, at this visit, all was satisfactory. However, perhaps the acute episode which resulted could have been picked up by a visit from other healthcare staff between CPN visits – or do we need to increase their frequency? I felt bad that Mrs A was admitted as I am aware that this often causes distress, and it made Mrs A upset.
4. **Analysis**: In your analysis, consider what might have helped or hindered the event. You also have the opportunity here to compare your experience with the literature you have read. This can act as a good way of bringing theory and experience together.	Being honest with Mrs A that I was disappointed that she felt the community services had let her down was important to ensuring we could continue to have a therapeutic relationship. Helping clients to learn practical strategies to effectively manage chronic conditions is one of the goals of therapeutic relationships (Arnold and Boggs 2016).
5. **Conclusion**: In your conclusion, it is important to acknowledge: whether you could have done anything else; what you have learned from the experience; consider	With the care plan that was in place there were no omissions from Mrs A's care. However, perhaps with hindsight Mrs A needed the support of more frequent visits or telephone calls between visits. Following the multidisciplinary team

Table 6.2 (Continued)

whether you could you have responded in a different way. If you are talking about a positive experience, discuss whether you would do the same again to ensure a positive outcome. Also, consider if there is anything you could change to improve things even further. If the incident was negative, tell your reader how you could have avoided it happening and also how you could make sure it doesn't happen again.	meeting, I discussed with Mrs A ways to support her in the future as I wished to continue to have a positive therapeutic relationship with her. She felt follow-up conversations would be a good way forward, and often feels differently prior to an acute episode. Advice at this point in time would be good for Mrs A and the team to prevent future hospital admissions.
6. **Action plan**: Action plans sum up anything you need to know and do to improve for next time. Perhaps you feel that you need to learn about something or attend some training. Within your healthcare setting, who could you ask for further advice or suggestions? What can you do so you will be better equipped to cope with a similar event?	Management of long-term caseload patients was discussed with my team leader and also as part of my clinical supervision. This has led to me feeling supported through the episode and allows the provision of telephone follow-ups between visits – at the instigation of the service user, where appropriate – thus avoiding the distress of admission to hospital.

Another reflective model you may be familiar with is the Driscoll (2007) or, as it is more commonly known, the 'What' Model of Reflection. An example using the Driscoll Model of Reflection is given next in Table 6.3 (with names changed to protect the patient's identity).

Table 6.3 An example of written reflection using the Driscoll Model of Reflection

What?	Mrs C was admitted to the care home where I am a registered nurse.
This stage is about describing the event you have chosen to return to: • What happened? • What did I see/do? • What did others do? • What was my reaction?	On admission, Mrs C appeared anxious and apprehensive. All staff welcomed Mrs C and, using verbal and non-verbal communication, I tried to make her feel welcome and reassure her that her preferences would be met.

(Continued)

Table 6.3 (Continued)

	My reaction was that this lady was very much out of her comfort zone and the huge step of moving from her family home to residential care was an emotional event. I wondered how we could make this transition easier for Mrs C and others. It was sad to see Mrs C visibly upset and worried.
So What? This stage is about analysing and making sense of your feelings and observations about the event. • What did I feel before/during/after the event? • What were the effects of what I did/did not do? • What have I noticed about my behaviour in practice? • What did I feel before/during/after the event?	My behaviour in practice was that I always make an effort to deliver the most person-centred care I can. However, on the day in question, the home had been really busy. We were short of two carers and, as a result, some of her preferences weren't met. I heard the carers saying they had no time to give her a bath, so she would just have to get a wash down instead. I didn't challenge this with them because, even though I knew Mrs C was anxious about living in the home and changes to her preferences, I knew we wouldn't be able to wash all of our patients in the way they had requested that day. This made me feel uncomfortable, but I had to prioritize the care being delivered.
Now What? This stage is about learning from the event, your proposed actions, and changes to your practice. • How could I modify my practice? • What support do I need to help me 'action'? • The results of my reflections? • Where can I get more information? • What are the implications for others?	I have learned that I should have challenged the carers to see if I could help support their workload and ensure Mrs C had a bath. I could also have explained to Mrs C that we were short-staffed, and that she could have a bath later in the day or check she was happy to have a wash instead. I have discussed this incident with my manager because Mrs C's family lodged a complaint when they realized she hadn't had a bath. I also want to make sure I share these reflections with the carers so they realize the impact of not giving Mrs C a bath had on her emotional well-being as a new resident within the home.
Are there any development needs that could be included in your PDP?	I would like to learn more about time management and communication to help me deal with situations like this better in the future.

As mentioned previously, it is a personal choice to choose which model you utilize. Other models are available, such as Johns' Model of Structured Reflection (Johns 2000), Boud's Triangular Representation Model of Reflection (Boud et al. 1985) and the Atkins and Murphy Model (Atkins and Murphy 1993). The most important aspect is that you choose something you are comfortable with which has personal appeal, as well as being clear and coherent (Nicol and Dosser 2016).

Facilitated reflection

Facilitated reflection is where you are guided by either a tool or an individual. It is particularly effective because it:

● Acts as a catalyst to think differently.
● Enhances motivation that may falter during everyday experiences.
● Assists a move from anxiety into positive energy for action.
● Addresses the gap between actual and desirable practice.
● Promotes deeper and critical levels of reflection.
● Challenges participants to respond differently in the practice situation.
● Supports staff to act on their insights with integrity.
● Supports staff morale during difficult times.
● Enables supervisees to be heard and re-energized.

(Helen and Douglas House 2015)

Facilitated reflection may involve multiple members of the multidisciplinary team which can provide more depth within the reflective process. In addition, the value of having different professionals discuss an issue or event is that they can provide an alternative view which encourages deeper reflection and thought.

Pitfalls to avoid when starting reflection

● You put it off!! Try to set aside some time to start reflecting, with a view to incorporating this into your practice.
● You assume reflection is simple. As mentioned earlier it takes practice, and you may change the model you are using – so don't give up!

- You describe too much. Nurses can be very descriptive, but what you are trying to do is learn from the reflection, so the description is to 'set the scene'.
- You make judgements about what has happened instead of describing your feelings about an event. Remember: it is your reflection, and this is where the rich learning will come to fruition.
- You do not ask for help. You do not have to undertake this activity alone, so get others involved so you can learn together.

Recording reflections for revalidation

Recording your reflections in writing is the last step of the process, and you are required to record a minimum of five written reflections on your CPD and/or practice-related feedback and/or an event or experience in your practice and how this relates to the Code (NMC 2015e). You may choose to write a reflection based on a combination of these – for example, if you receive feedback from an incident or event in your practice you may undertake some CPD to address this and want to include this as a reflective account. The purpose of this requirement is to encourage registrants to engage in reflective practice and make changes or improvements to their practice based on what they have learned. The NMC guidelines must be followed at all times to ensure this meets the most up-to-date NMC revalidation requirements. The NMC have developed a mandatory template with key headings that you must use. You have to fill in a page for each of your reflections, ensuring you do not include any information that might identify a specific patient or service user. No reflective model is specified, so it is up to you which one you want to use. Or, you can populate the headings in the template without using a specific model at all.

You must then discuss these reflections as part of a reflective discussion with another NMC registrant and show these to your confirmer. To help with the discussion it may be useful for you to read the reflective discussion chapter of this book.

The NMC website must be checked on a regular basis to ensure you are using the most up-to-date guidance, templates and forms, but the broad areas that are required are included in Box 6.2.

Box 6.2: Areas you should cover in your reflective accounts

Reflective account:

- Describe the nature of the CPD activity and/or practice-related feedback and/or event or experience in your practice.
- What did you learn from the CPD activity and/or practice related feedback and/or event or experience in your practice?
- How did you change or improve your practice as a result?
- How is this relevant to the Code (NMC 2015a)? You are required to select one or more themes from the Code. These include: Prioritize People, Practise Effectively, Preserve Safety, Promote Professionalism and Trust.

(NMC 2015e)

Summary

This chapter has explored the terminology in relation to reflection and described some of the common models. Readers are advised to make it personal to them and be aware that practice is necessary to undertake this successfully. Within practice there are many opportunities to reflect, and this can be done as an individual or incorporating a team approach. It is recommended that this becomes part of routine practice rather than waiting for when it is necessary to do this to satisfy the NMC revalidation requirements.

Key points

- Reflection is a valuable tool you can use when learning more about yourself and your practice.
- Reflection can take place on your own or with others – it is your choice. However, in order to meet the NMC revalidation requirements you must complete five individual reflective accounts.
- Consider the models described in this chapter and choose one that suits your needs. This may change over time.
- Writing your reflections as close to the time of the incident or event as possible will help you develop your practice and meet the NMC revalidation requirements.

Reflective discussion

Introduction

The NMC require every registrant to have one reflective conversation as part of their three-yearly revalidation cycle. You should already have gained a working understanding of reflection from the previous chapter. The aim of this chapter is to take you through the elements of an effective reflective discussion to support you to meet the NMC revalidation requirements. This discussion is a mandatory part of the revalidation model and every registrant will be required to have a reflective discussion, with another NMC registrant, prior to confirmation.

This chapter will cover this activity from both perspectives; having a reflective conversation as a registrant due to revalidate and also as a reflective discussion partner. To make the most of your reflective discussion this chapter will also give you a brief tour of interpersonal and communication issues as they relate to the revalidation process. This will also help you understand how you can use reflective discussions as part of a cycle of lifelong learning (see Chapter 4) and not just for the purposes of meeting the NMC revalidation requirements.

Learning objectives

By the end of this chapter you will be able to:

- Describe how to meet the NMC revalidation standard for a reflective discussion.
- Explain the role of communication in a reflective discussion.

- Discuss the benefits of a reflective discussion.
- Hold a reflective discussion.

Current NMC revalidation requirements

The NMC (NMC 2015c: 22) states that:

'You must have had a reflective discussion with another NMC registrant, covering your five written reflective accounts on your CPD and/or practice-related feedback and/or an event or experience in your practice and how this relates to the Code.'

Always refer to the NMC website for the most up-to-date revalidation guidance.

Reflective practice

Before we consider the reflective discussion you will need to have in order to revalidate, you should be clear about the concept behind 'reflective practice'. Reflective practice has been described as a self-regulating learning process where we assess our own thoughts and actions for the purpose of personal learning and development. This is an intuitive process in that reflective practice often occurs without thinking about it and remains a successful way of developing healthcare professionals (Nath et al. 2014) (see Chapter 6 for more information on reflection).

Donald Schön is credited with making a significant contribution to the theory and practice of reflective practice. It is worth reading Schön's definition below, in particular the way he describes reflection as the way we learn through constructing our own meanings and perspectives, within individual contexts and experiences (Masella 2007; Tsang 2010).

> The practitioner allows himself to experience surprise, puzzlement, or confusion in a situation which he finds uncertain or unique. He reflects on the phenomenon before him, and on the prior understandings which have been implicit in his behaviour.

He carries out an experiment which serves to generate both a new understanding of the phenomenon and a change in the situation.

(Schön 1983: 68)

Time Out

Once you have read the definition above, ask yourself if this resonates with how you view reflective practice. Depending on your thoughts it may be helpful to review Chapter 6 again.

As part of your ongoing personal and professional development it is useful to reflect on your practice with another registrant. We all learn best in different ways (as explored in Chapter 3). For example, you may be primarily an auditory or visual learner, and some people may gain more benefit from discussing their reflections than from writing them. You should approach the conversation as an opportunity to learn and look for the benefit it can give you for your practice.

A reflective conversation can enhance professional understanding and support deeper learning through the discussion of professional issues (Kolyva 2015). Reflective discussions often take place informally as part of everyday practice, and this may happen either in isolation or as part of a team. You may have someone you reflect with on a regular basis; this will be someone you already trust or have a rapport with. You may also reflect with many different healthcare professionals; however, for the purposes of meeting the NMC revalidation requirements you must have your reflective conversation with another NMC registrant – either a nurse or midwife (NMC 2015e).

Having a reflective discussion

The first step is familiarizing yourself with the most up-to-date NMC revalidation guidance available from the NMC website (https://www.nmc.org.uk). Then it is for you to decide who the most appropriate reflective discussion partner should be, remembering they must be an NMC registrant (NMC 2015e) (see Figure 7.1). This means they must be on the NMC register with a current NMC PIN number and cannot have been removed from the register for any reason. For example, they cannot have been suspended or struck off by the NMC or have a lapsed registration due to retirement or voluntary removal (NMC 2015e).

If your line manager is an NMC registrant then the reflective discussion can be held with them at the same time as confirmation, if you wish. However, if your line manager is not an NMC registrant then the conversation will need to be held with another NMC registrant before confirmation can take place (see Chapter 9 for more on confirmation).

If you do not wish to have your reflective discussion with your line manager at the same time as confirmation – either because they are

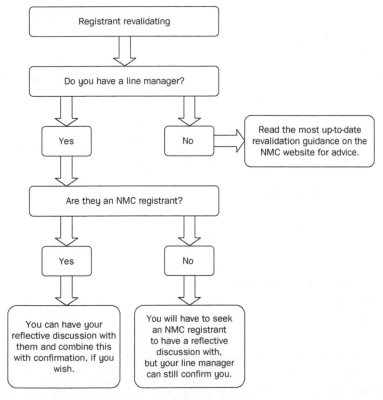

Figure 7.1 Choosing your reflective discussion partner

not an NMC registrant or because you do not wish to have a reflective discussion with them – you will have to find another NMC registrant to have the reflective discussion with.

Choosing a reflective discussion partner

You may want to discuss your choice of reflective discussion partner with your line manager or with your peers; however, this remains your individual decision. The reflective partner you choose could be a registrant you work with on a regular basis or someone from within a professional or specialist network, depending on your scope of practice – for example, you may have access to an independent midwifery group or military defence service nurse network. You may choose a registrant you already have a professional relationship with, such as a critical companion, coach, clinical supervisor or mentor (see Chapter 8).

Time Out

Consider the qualities of a reflective discussion partner. What attributes would you want them to possess, and why?

Some of the qualities of a desirable 'reflective discussion partner' you might have considered are listed below.

They are a registrant who is:

- Approachable.
- Non-judgemental.
- Open.
- A good, active listener.
- Respectful.
- Curious.
- Compassionate.
- A challenger in a positive constructive way.
- Kind.
- Empathetic.
- Supportive.

It's possible you will have identified several registrants within your professional sphere who possess these qualities, but it is important that you consider whether you would be comfortable discussing your practice with this registrant. You will want to take some time and consider this carefully as not every registrant may be suitable. As a professional you should consider any conflicts of interest, and it is not appropriate to select a close friend or a member of your family (NMC 2015e).

The reflective discussion partner must be currently practising as either a registered nurse or midwife and they should have an understanding of your practice (NMC 2015e). Your reflective discussion partner does not have to be on the same part of the register as you and it does not matter if they are in a similar position or in one more senior or junior to you. However, if you choose someone junior to you this may limit their ability to challenge your practice. This position may also be subject to local guidance, so check any local policies for the most up-to-date information in relation to this. The most important consideration is that your reflective discussion partner is someone you can have a meaningful reflective discussion with.

You can have your reflective discussion at any point in the 12 months prior to your revalidation date. This will allow time for you to plan when this will take place and, if possible, to align this to existing appraisal processes; however, if you do this then part of the appraisal meeting must centre on the content of your written reflective accounts. This discussion must focus on your reflections and how they relate to the Code (NMC 2015a) while also giving you the opportunity to highlight any changes or improvements to your practice. This approach is designed to encourage a culture of sharing and improvement across the nursing and midwifery professions, and reduce professional isolation (Kolyva 2015).

Pause for Thought

Written reflections can come from multiple sources and you may have discussed these with several people. However, you need to have your reflective discussion with **ONE** registered nurse or midwife to include the content of all **FIVE** reflective accounts.

Preparation

Once you have identified your reflective discussion partner it is important that you prepare for the discussion. You must have completed at least five written reflective accounts, prior to your reflective discussion meeting, in accordance with the most up-to-date information and templates from the NMC (see also Chapter 6). It is advisable to reread your reflective accounts to refresh your memory prior to the reflective discussion meeting as these will have been collated over a three-year period. When you read your reflective accounts it is worth considering what your feelings and thoughts were at the time. These may have changed, and you may have built further on what you have learned, so it is a good idea to make notes about your reflections so you can discuss these more fully during your reflective discussion. You may also realize how your practice has improved over your revalidation period by reflecting on what you have learned. This is something to raise at your reflective discussion meeting for further discussion with your partner. It is also worth sending these reflective accounts to your reflective discussion partner in advance of the meeting as this will also give them the opportunity to fully read and reflect on these, which should lead to a more meaningful discussion.

You can produce these reflections either by writing them on paper or in an electronic format; you must ensure that when sharing this information with your partner in advance that they are being kept in a safe place. Although the information in them must be anonymized, they may still contain confidential reflections about situations or your feelings (see Chapter 10 for more information).

Before we consider elements like the environment in which you carry out your discussion, tips for helpful communication, and techniques for reflective questioning and listening, we will first define the role of the reflective discussion partner.

The role of reflective discussion partner

The role of the reflective discussion partner is to discuss the registrant's reflective accounts with them and use this discussion to guide them to explore beyond the problems and outcomes identified in their reflective accounts. They should be able to appropriately challenge the underlying beliefs, values, assumptions, relevance and alternatives to the reflections. Any NMC registrant can take on the role of reflective discussion partner; however, some registrants will feel more comfortable with this role than others, especially if they have had some experience as a mentor or coach. If you are approached to be a reflective discussion partner then you can discuss this more fully with the registrant before you decide whether to take on this role or not. There is no requirement for you to receive any special training, but you will need to prepare for your role by understanding the purpose of the reflective discussion, which you can do by reading the most up-to-date NMC guidance available from their website (https://www.nmc.org.uk).

Pause for Thought

Every NMC registrant will have to go through the revalidation process – including you! So consider if any of your peers would be a good source of support if you are asked to be a reflective discussion partner.

Your reflective partner should be someone with the attributes identified earlier in this chapter. They should be sensitive and able to provide emotional support, if required, because the reflections may uncover sensitive issues. It is worth remembering that a reflection may evoke expected as well as unexpected feelings and emotions. So it is important that, as a reflective discussion partner, you are prepared for this and can respond appropriately. If necessary, you may need to take a break during the meeting and resume the discussions later.

The reflective discussion partner is responsible for enabling effective two-way communication to allow the registrant to discuss their reflective accounts more fully, and it is important to allow the registrant revalidating to 'own' the discussion. Check with the registrant that they are happy to discuss their reflections with you and allow them to decide the order; this may be done in date order or even in themes. You must also ensure no individuals are named or can be identified during the discussion, and this includes both colleagues and service users, clients or patients (NMC 2015e).

It would also be helpful for you to revisit and understand the most commonly used models of reflection such as Gibbs (1988) or Driscoll (2007) as you may wish to use these to guide the discussion (for more information on these, see Chapter 6). It is also a good idea for you both to have a copy of the Code (NMC 2015a) to hand during the discussion in case you want to refer to it.

How to begin?

The most effective two-way communication takes place face-to-face, so it is worth remembering that if meeting in person is not possible you should have your reflective discussion using a video conference or similar system.

When beginning your reflective discussion it is important to build rapport, if necessary – this will usually depend on how well you know the registrant. It is normal to begin a conversation with a short general discussion to break the ice; this might be in relation to what they have been doing that day, or a recent event such as a holiday or weekend. However, when you start the reflective discussion it is important to ensure you focus on the written reflective accounts, what the registrant has learned, and how this learning links to their practice and the Code (NMC 2015a). It can be easy to digress, especially if you have a good relationship with each other, but try to be aware of this and get back on track when possible.

Having a reflective discussion

A reflective discussion must be planned and should take place when there is time set aside to have the discussion. It is important, if you have your reflective discussions over the three years leading up to your revalidation date as part of the appraisal process, that one person then has the final reflective discussion with you, covering all five reflective accounts (NMC 2015e). As discussed earlier in this chapter, this may or may not take place at the same time as the confirmation discussion (see also Chapter 9).

You must set aside an appropriate time for this conversation to take place – for example, not when you are in charge of the shift or have an appointment that you have to rush off to. There is no set time advised for this to take place, so discuss this between you and your reflective discussion partner in advance of the meeting and gain agreement on this. It is always best to allow more time than you may need as you want to ensure you have enough time for a quality discussion to take place.

Environment

The discussion should be held in an open environment, focus on individual experiences and provide another professional's perspective (Kolyva 2015). The reflective discussion is a confidential conversation and must be held in an appropriate setting because the physical environment can influence effective communication both positively and negatively (Westwick 2013). The discussion should be held in a safe, appropriate area, away from distractions where noise and interruptions are minimized. Although this is a professional discussion, some people may feel intimidated or reluctant to speak if the setting is too formal, so you may choose to hold this in a slightly more informal environment to encourage a more open discussion (Thompson 2009). For example, imagine how you would feel having the discussion in a clinic room compared to an office. The environment you choose can influence individual feelings, so the registrant should ideally choose where and when this discussion takes place.

The room itself should be bright and comfortable because temperature and comfort can affect concentration (Thompson 2009). You should also be sitting on chairs of a similar height as each other because it can cause a perceived power imbalance if someone is on a higher or lower chair than you (Thompson 2009). This discussion should be a positive opportunity for both the registrant and the reflective discussion partner to learn and share professional experiences. In this situation you are peers and equals, and you should both ensure the discussion is held in this way.

Interpersonal space

You should be aware of the feelings associated with interpersonal space when having your reflective discussion. We often feel anxious if someone enters our interpersonal space at a distance we are not comfortable with; this is influenced by culture, gender and personality, and these distances cannot be completely predicted or measured (Patterson and Edinger 2014).

When we refer to the space around us we generally have four levels or zones of interpersonal spaces (see Figure 7.2). These are:

1   Intimate.
2   Personal.
3   Social.
4   Public.

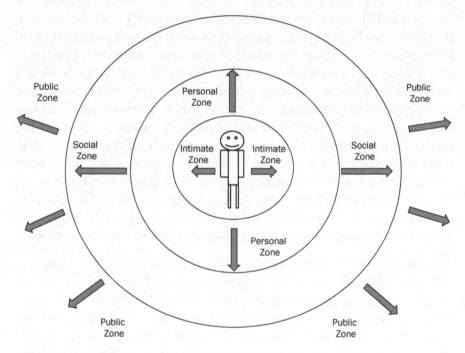

Figure 7.2 Interpersonal zones

Table 7.1 Approximate distances for the zones of interpersonal space

Interpersonal zone	Approximate distance	Examples
Intimate	Touch up to 46cm away.	Closeness, such as a physical examination.
Personal	46cm to 1.2m.	1:1 conversation.
Social	1.2m to approximately 3.7m.	Conversation with a group.
Public	3.7m outwards.	Giving a talk to a group of people or behaviour with strangers.

As you can see from the distances in Table 7.1, the 'public zone' makes it difficult to have an effective two-way conversation and the 'intimate zone' can feel very uncomfortable if we are not familiar with the person. You should therefore consider your seating position when having your reflective conversation as you both want to feel comfortable. Ideally, you should be in reasonably close proximity to each other, at a distance equivalent of the 'personal zone' (Rosdahl and Kowalski 2008).

Time Out

What approximate distances are your intimate, personal, social and public zones?

How does this change, based on the type of communication encounter and the nature of the relationship you have with the person with whom you are communicating?

What alters this feeling and how comfortable does this feel?

You may find that you want to move your position closer or further away from someone when you are speaking to them. This feeling will often be altered by the relationship you have with the person (Rosdahl and Kowalski 2008). As healthcare professionals we often operate in the 'intimate' zone with our patients or clients, and this is often not thought about in the same way. When communicating with others you want to consider not only the physical environment and proximity, but also the way in which we communicate; this applies to both the registrant and the reflective discussion partner.

Communication

There are many definitions of what communication is, as humans we cannot stop ourselves from communicating (McCabe and Timmins 2013). One definition of communication is:

> 'Communication involves the reciprocal process in which messages are sent or received between two or more people.'
>
> (Balzer-Riley 2011: 6)

Another is:

> 'A series of messages – information – which can be sent out to other people and messages which you received from them, through seeing, hearing or touching one another.'
>
> (Petrie 1997: 6)

However, it is difficult to precisely define the dynamic, complex and continuous nature of communication. There are many different models which aim to explain this, and you may be familiar with these already (McCabe and Timmins 2013).

Models of communication

Linear or transmission model (Miller and Nicholson 1976)

The sender intentionally transmits a message to the receiver; this message contains verbal and/or non-verbal information, and the sender usually knows the information has been received or interpreted through feedback (see Figure 7.3). This is a linear process, and is rarely an effective method of communication; it has several limitations in that it doesn't take account of other factors which can influence the communication process (McCabe and Timmins 2013).

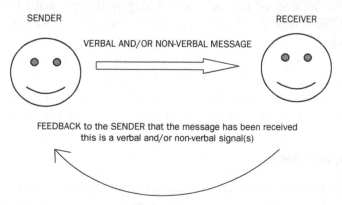

Figure 7.3 Linear or transmission model

Example

Marie Brown is a senior nurse. She is presenting her findings on an audit she has undertaken to her team. When she tells them the main findings she notices they are nodding their heads in agreement (non-verbal feedback), and one of her staff asks a question (verbal feedback). This is the transmission model.

Circular transactional model (Bateson 1979)

This model is a more fluid transactional model of communication which builds upon the simple theory explained in the linear model and expands it to include the principle that we send and receive communication simultaneously (Barnlund 2008) (see Figure 7.4). This is viewed as a two-way interactive process, and takes into account the factors which may influence the communication process. This has been described as a way of generating meaning by sending messages and receiving feedback within physical and psychological contexts where the participants alternate their positions from sender to receiver (McCabe and Timmins 2013).

Example

Ani Noon is a nurse practitioner. She is conducting a reflective discussion with one of the staff nurses. As the nurse describes the feedback detailed in the reflective account, Ani is actively listening and processing what she is saying and responding using non-verbal and verbal communication. They are simultaneously interpreting each other's verbal and non-verbal messages, and the communication flow is fluid.

The transactional model represents most conversations we have.

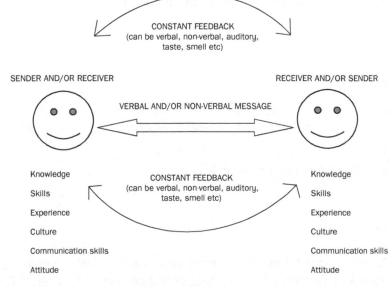

Figure 7.4 Circular transactional model

The two main types of communication referred to are verbal and non-verbal. Although these are split into distinctive categories, they are actually inextricably linked, and one cannot exist without the other (Burgoon et al. 2016).

Non-verbal

Non-verbal communication is the way we communicate without words, and can be a controlled response or automatic behaviour. The difference between what is said and how we interpret what has been said is through non-verbal communication – 'body language', as it is more commonly known.

Actions such as body posture, eye contact, facial expressions, closeness/touch are all types of non-verbal communication which have been defined as 'a code which is to be interpreted' (Thompson 2009). Some non-verbal communication is automatic in that we will respond in a learned way – for example, when we smell something unpleasant we pull a face and may shrivel our noses up. We may react automatically to a number of situations, but you should be self-aware of your non-verbal behaviour and how this communicates a message to the receiver. This message can be interpreted in many different ways, and it is sometimes said 'you can read people like a book'; however, this is very rarely a true statement (Burgoon et al. 2016).

Time Out

Consider the non-verbal communication in Table 7.2 and what it would mean to you if you saw someone displaying this during a conversation?

How would you feel?

What else might influence your feelings?

You may have considered the following:

● A smile may mean that someone is happy, but depending on how you interpret this, a smile could convey a feeling of falseness or insincerity.

Table 7.2 Non-verbal communication and what it means to you

Non-verbal communication	What would this mean to you?
Smile	
Avoiding eye contact	
Yawn	
Standing close by	
Looking straight into your eyes	
Head nod	
Pause	

- Avoiding eye contact may mean that you are hiding something, or that you just don't feel comfortable talking, but this can also be normal behaviour for some people who find it difficult to look straight at someone.
- A yawn can be a sign of boredom. It can also be interpreted in different ways – the person may simply be tired or disinterested.
- Looking straight into someone's eyes can feel intimidating or intimate; it can also mean someone has your full attention. If you stare at someone for longer than three seconds then they can feel uncomfortable or even threatened; this has the same effect as invading someone's intimate zone or space (Patterson and Edinger 2014).
- A head nod can be perceived as a positive gesture or a sign of agreement.
- A pause can be a good thing because it can allow the person time to respond or think, but if the pause is too long it can make the person feel uncomfortable.

These are just examples of the ways non-verbal gestures can be interpreted differently and how they may make you feel. However, you will also have recognized that the way you interpret them is influenced by a number of factors. These may have included the environment, the context, the person, your relationship with them, how you are feeling, and any verbal communication (Burgoon et al. 2016). However, this list is not exhaustive and there are many aspects to non-verbal communication including the various codes or cues, the message it may convey, the purpose of the non-verbal communication and the way in which all of this can be interpreted. It has been estimated that between 66 per cent and 93 per cent of all communication is non-verbal (Birdwhistell 1955; Mehrabian and Ferris 1967).

Time Out

If you want to read more about communication then you can read any of the books which have been referred to. You may want to access further learning in relation to this topic by doing a literature search or speaking to colleagues.

Remember: reading this book, and any further reading or learning you do, can be counted and logged as CPD for revalidation purposes.

Why is non-verbal communication important for a reflective discussion?

The use of appropriate non-verbal communication can support an effective reflective discussion. Gestures such as a head nod, warm facial expression, open posture and eye contact can reinforce your genuineness and encourage the registrant to be more open. This can also make the registrant feel at ease, particularly in relation to emotional aspects of the discussion.

Verbal communication

It is important to consider verbal communication when facilitating a reflective discussion because the relationship between language and meaning is not straightforward. The English language has millions of different words, many of which have different meanings depending on the context in which they are used.

Context of language

"Run"

This word sounds the same and is pronounced in the same way, but has many different meanings. For example:

He *runs* a successful aesthetic clinic (means manages).
She gave me a *run* through of the shift pattern (means showing or describing briefly).

I *run* home after a night shift (means moving your legs quickly – not easy after a night shift!).

We have had a *run* of home births (means a succession of similar events).

We *run* an out-of-hours service in this area (means offering a service).

It is important that you not only consider the language and meaning of what you say, but also the speed, pitch, tone and volume you use. You will want to vary the tone of what you say, keeping the pitch even and volume low, as this discussion must be a two-way conversation which is supportive and non-threatening. You may have experience of having a reflective conversation before, so draw on what you learned and use this for reflection purposes.

Time Out

Say the word 'Revalidation' in a:

Silly voice
Laughing
Angrily
Sarcastically
Shout it out
Squeak it out

How did it make you feel when you heard it being said in different ways? What did you do to your voice to evoke those feelings?

How could this influence the way you communicate during your reflective discussion?

The seven key principles of effective communication adapted from the work of Cutlip et al. (2006) are that all communication should be:

1   Clear
2   Concise
3   Concrete

4   Correct
5   Coherent
6   Complete
7   Courteous

It is helpful to keep these in mind when you are having your reflective discussion, both as the registrant and the reflective discussion partner.

Barriers to effective communication

Time Out

Consider the main barriers to effective communication. What are these and how can you minimize them during your reflective discussion?

Some of the barriers to effective communication you may have identified are: language, emotions, poor listening, lack of interest, physical barriers, attitude and ambiguity. This list is not exhaustive. Each of these barriers you have identified can each be minimized by understanding and practising the principles of good communication and reflecting on previous conversations you may have had.

Reflective listening

To engage effectively with reflective listening, you must be a good active listener, as this reassures and encourages the registrant to speak freely and openly. Active listening is a way of ensuring the person you are communicating with knows you are listening to them and that you seek to understand what they mean (Burgoon et al. 2016). You should focus fully on the speaker and show you are interested, and be objective as you are not there to pass judgement or make decisions for the registrant. Avoid interrupting, jumping to conclusions or making assumptions. Acknowledging the registrant's feelings, it is important to show you value what is being said. Listening with empathy is not just about hearing – it is about understanding where the other person is coming from.

Reflective questioning

As the reflective discussion partner, it is best practice to view the five reflective accounts in advance; this will allow you to read these and make any observations prior to the meeting. This also allows you to prepare some specific questions and prompts, which may be particularly useful if you are new to reflective discussions.

Planning your discussion in this way may also have a negative side; it has the potential to quash or limit the discussion, dominate any discussion, or perhaps even make you lead any thoughts the registrant may have. The purpose of the discussion is not to question the registrant in an intrusive way (always use non-threatening language) but to support and encourage deeper reflection and discussion on what they have reflected on, how this learning has linked to the Code (NMC 2015a), and what impact it has had on their practice (NMC 2015e).

When considering the questions, you may consider asking probing or open questions as these may help you to explore knowledge, skills, experience, attitudes, beliefs and values more deeply. You must ensure that you are able to work with whatever ideas, thoughts, feelings and issues that may arise. By being responsive to these feelings you will maximize the quality and effectiveness of this discussion.

Types of questions

Table 7.3 describes each type of question you may consider asking as a reflective discussion partner.

Responses

When you ask different questions, and in particular, probing questions, you must be prepared for different types of answers and use your communication skills effectively to support the registrant. Effective two-way communication can be challenging, especially when dealing with feelings both as a registrant and as the reflective discussion partner. Failing to take both sets of feelings into account can cause problems during the discussion. It is important to acknowledge your own feelings; you will need a degree of objectivity and

Table 7.3 Questions to ask as a reflection partner

Type of question	Example
Open: This is a useful type of question that allows the person to answer fully and encourages more involvement in the conversation.	'Tell me about how you felt when this happened'.
Closed: This type of question usually requires one or two words and often a yes or no answer. These questions can be used as a way of clarifying or getting a direct answer.	'So you felt angry?'
Leading: This type of question is not usually useful – it tends to be viewed as manipulative.	'Did you feel angry when this happened?'
Funnelling: In this type of approach you start with closed questions, then open questions, or vice versa, which can allow the conversation to feel more relaxed.	'Tell me about the feedback you received.' 'So what about the email you read?' 'How did that make you feel?' 'So you said that made you feel angry?' 'How did you resolve this situation?' 'So you feel this is now resolved?'
Clarification: This type of question may be probing, or you may clarify by summarizing what the person has said.	'Can you tell me a bit more about why you felt angry when that happened?'

detachment to be able to do this. It is also important to recognize distress and offer support to the registrant if required.

Effective questioning is a skill which develops over time. It is worth asking for feedback from the registrant you have undertaken the reflective discussion with, as you can learn from this experience (see Chapter 5). You may also wish to reflect on this experience for your own revalidation evidence, which may prompt you to undertake some CPD to develop your communication skills, or you may use the feedback as part of your revalidation evidence.

Dealing with difficult issues

Registrants may feel you are challenging them when you ask questions about their reflections. This can naturally make some people feel uncomfortable, so it is important you are aware of the need for regular breaks and have the ability to notice if the conversation is upsetting or causing conflict. By questioning the registrant about their reflective accounts you must bear in mind this may be interpreted as questioning them about their practice. At the start of the conversation it is worth having a brief discussion about what the reflective discussion is about, and what it is not about, to ensure you both understand the purpose of the conversation. You might not be the right reflective discussion partner, or either of you may not be in the right frame of mind to have the discussion. You must act as a professional at all times, and if you feel unable to continue your reflective discussion for any reason then you should make sure you are able to have a professional conversation about this (NMC 2015a).

Top tips to facilitate an effective discussion

- Make direct eye contact.
- Stay in tune with your own and others' body language.
- Use non-verbal signals that match up with your words. Consider what you have read regarding body language – e.g. smile, open posture etc.
- Adjust your non-verbal signals according to the context.
- Use body language to convey positive feelings.
- Practise it with a smile.
- Use standard terminology – try not to use abbreviations or colloquialisms.
- Use verbal tone, speed and pitch to communicate appropriately.
- Request and provide clarification if needed.
- Use straight, clear statements.
- Stay focused.
- Listen carefully.
- Be open if you feel upset or you want the discussion to end.
- Ask for feedback to allow improvement.

Documenting the reflective discussion

Many registrants will undertake aspects of reflective practice, including discussing their reflections with other registrants, but this may not be done formally and they may not make a record of these conversations. Note taking is an important part of the discussion to ensure an accurate record of the conversation can be made on the appropriate NMC form, including suggestions for future actions or objectives. This is detailed further in Chapter 10.

You must ensure that the NMC registrant with whom you had your reflective discussion signs the most up-to-date NMC form. This can be a physical or electronic signature.

The type of information recorded is likely to include their name, NMC PIN, address and email, as well as the date you had the discussion and a summary of what you discussed. See the NMC website for the most up-to-date form which must be completed.

Benefits to the registrant and the reflective discussion partner

As a registrant, reflective practice is an integral part of your development and enhances professionalism by encouraging you to reflect on the standard of care provided, no matter what role you are in. Developing your self-awareness as a practitioner contributes to public safety because it allows you to take ownership of this process. It also offers a real opportunity to reflect on The Code (NMC 2015a) and how it is used in practice. As a reflective discussion partner you can learn a lot from having a reflective discussion. Your role is to support the registrant, but you may also gain some deeper understanding of the issues raised and may choose to log this for your own CPD or reflect on this independently.

Engaging in additional reflective conversations outwith the minimum revalidation requirements, as part of your personal and professional development, will enhance your practice. You can undertake this with as many different professionals as you wish, and may also choose to log this as CPD for revalidation purposes.

Summary

This chapter has encouraged readers to explore different aspects of having a reflective discussion, including effective planning, the value of questioning and reflective listening, as well as highlighting the importance of effective two-way verbal and non-verbal communication. Having a reflective discussion can be a valuable learning experience for both the registrant and the reflective discussion partner, and can lead to further learning. Although a reflective discussion is a requirement of revalidation, this may be of use throughout your career, not just to meet the NMC revalidation requirements but also to encourage personal development through reflective conversations.

Key points

- Read the most up-to-date guidance, tools and templates from the NMC.
- Make sure you select an appropriate reflective discussion partner.
- Ensure the environment is conducive to an effective discussion.
- Good two-way communication is key.
- Make sure you record the notes from the discussion to allow you to meet the NMC revalidation requirements.
- Consider having reflective discussions as part of your day-to-day practice.

8 Supportive relationships

This chapter is aimed at providing ideas to make use of the support and expertise of others within your practice as you seek to take advantage of learning opportunities, acquire and take action on feedback, and discuss your career progression. Many routes for advice and information will be available to you, but you may not be making the most of these at this moment in time in your normal daily practice. Purposefully developing supportive relationships with other professionals will have several benefits, and this will include invaluable support through the revalidation process. This chapter will help you identify those who can support you in this way. In this chapter there are many examples which are aimed at helping you to consider what relationships may be of use, not only for revalidation but also for your career and personal development. This may also assist you in considering suitable colleagues who can take on the role of reflective discussion partner and/or confirmer (also see Chapters 7 and 9).

Learning objectives

By the end of the chapter you will be able to:

- Describe the types of supportive relationships that are available.
- Assess and explore which supportive relationships will be beneficial to your practice.
- Consider developing your network and influencing others.
- Identify any professional relationships to support you with revalidation.

Types of support roles

Support and encouragement can have a huge impact for an effective learning environment to flourish, and you will want to consider which individuals can provide this. Within healthcare, supportive learning relationships can be formed in a variety of contexts, and those who have different roles can be used to support you. These support roles can be classified as informal, formal, and regulatory as shown in Table 8.1.

This chapter will start by describing roles which you will no doubt be familiar with in practice – e.g. mentor and preceptor. The chapter will then evaluate ways to expand your networks to further develop relationships within the workplace or elsewhere to help support you to meet the revalidation requirements.

Mentors

Jasper (2006) describes mentors as usually having a supervisory and assessment component to their role where they are involved in enabling the development of the 'student' in becoming a safe and

Table 8.1 Types of roles to support learning

Role type	Definition	Examples
Informal	This is usually outside of a formal education context. It can be led by the individual, line manager or peers and include formal, informal, planned or ad hoc support.	Induction 'buddy' for new members of staff. Shadowing. Critical companionship.
Formal	This type of role tends to support more defined learning outcomes. Due to the nature of the role it will usually require some knowledge or preparation for both parties.	Clinical supervisor. Action learning. Mentorship role. Work-based supervisor for a course of study.
Regulatory	These often include individuals with a regulatory role or function within nursing practice who are expected to adhere to defined parameters.	The role of confirmer and reflective discussion partner as detailed in 'How to Revalidate with the NMC' (NMC 2015e). NMC sign-off mentor (NMC 2008c).

competent practitioner. She describes it as 'one likely to be of unequal status' with the person being mentored; in other words, there will be an experienced practitioner supervising a less experienced colleague. In relation to pre-registration nursing education the Standards for Learning and Assessment in Practice outline the requirements and specific outcomes for mentors, practice teachers and teachers within practice (NMC 2008c). The role of NMC mentor is a person who has the knowledge and skills to support and assess students in practice who are undertaking a pre-registration course that leads to registration or a recordable qualification on the register (NMC 2006d). You may have been mentored during your education and preparation for becoming a registered nurse or midwife, or indeed you may fulfil the role of mentor to pre-registration and other students within practice. Note that although a mentor is traditionally linked to a course or a new role, this is not exclusive.

There are other forms of mentors too that you can consider, and this is your chance to think about someone who has the skills, attributes or knowledge you wish to learn from. You may wish to discuss having a work-based mentor as part of your personal development plan which will have direct relevance to both your career and individual aspects for development – e.g. improving your confidence in multidisciplinary meetings. The advantage to agreeing this as part of your PDP is that you are more likely to get work-based support for this, and combining this with setting objectives means that both parties are clear on the aspects you wish to develop.

If you are choosing a mentor you may consider the following:

- Does this person have the skills and knowledge base that I wish to learn from? Will they be able to support my adult learning within practice?
- Is this person one I could get along with and trust? Building rapport and feeling comfortable and confident are key aspects of the relationship, as is a balance of support and challenge. Remember that the relationship is applicable to both parties and the mentor will learn and get positive experiences from being a mentor to you.
- Do they have time to dedicate to my needs? For example, think about the duration of support you expect to receive and the timing of meetings, or how frequent you expect them to be.

This will ensure both parties are clear on their roles and responsibilities.

- Take time to do some research regarding suitable individuals, and consider being brave and choosing a more senior member of staff. The benefits to involving more senior staff is that they may be able to give their varied experiences of events that you have not been exposed to, and may assist in developing opportunities for you to experience these events in a safe and supportive way.

Preceptors

Preceptorship has been identified as important in preparing newly registered nurses and midwives for the transition from student to practitioner. The Department of Health have developed a preceptorship framework to support this (Department of Health 2010). A preceptor is a registered practitioner, in this case either a nurse or midwife, who helps new registrants develop confidence and reinforces their knowledge and skills after their initial registration (NMC 2006). In a broader context, preceptors are defined by Mills et al. (2005) as experienced nurses who give formal feedback on the preceptee's performance to his or her supervisor or lecturer. They also state that this is a formal role assumed over a short period in addition to their defined clinical responsibilities. Registrants are often allocated a preceptor when they first qualify, and this is often a short-term supportive role until the practitioner feels more comfortable within that area of practice and is deemed competent.

Time Out

Who is available to support your learning in your area? For example, a practice teacher or educator?

Do you have a mentor or preceptor? Is this something you feel you want? Can you ask for this?

If you don't require a formal role such as mentorship or preceptorship, can you identify anybody within your practice who has the particular skills and attributes that can support your learning and development?

You may consider that neither mentorship nor preceptorship are appropriate supportive roles for you at this time; there are other relationships to consider which you may find more helpful such as coaching, clinical supervision and critical companionship, and these will be explored next.

Coaching

Coaching is a method of helping others to improve, develop, learn new skills, achieve aims and manage professional and personal challenges. Coaching commonly addresses attitudes, behaviours, and knowledge, as well as skills, and can also focus on physical and spiritual development too (Chapman 2010). Many organizations have networks of individuals who can provide coaching, and this service is often provided free of charge. Sometimes coaching is available from within the organization, but you may also be able to access a coach from a partner organization. The benefit of this is that you can receive coaching from someone with a different professional background – for example, business or management. This also means they are independent, which can result in a more valuable coaching experience because you may feel more comfortable discussing your personal goals.

Within coaching relationships a first meeting is usually conducted to check both parties are happy, often referred to as a 'chemistry' meeting. Following this, ways of working and what you wish the outcomes to be will be planned. Typically it can provide the following:

- Encourage career development and goal setting.
- Focus on personal development and how to achieve this.
- Promote self-awareness.
- Provide a safe space to explore all options for development.
- Offer a degree of challenge and support that is agreed.
- Encourage reflection in and on actions within the workplace.
- Offer feedback and support in relation to work issues.

A successful coaching relationship will typically involve defining goals through collaboration, good communication and interaction, involve mutual respect, understanding, and facilitate learning (Fielden et al. 2009). As with mentoring, the balance between challenge and support is essential for success. With modern technology, meeting face-to-face may not be required every time, and a telephone call, Skype call etc. can be used to maximize time for both parties. It has been shown to be an extremely effective method of supporting individuals to develop leadership behaviours (Thatch 2002) and this could be through self-awareness, reflection or focused learning.

Pause for Thought

Consider if having a coach would benefit your practice. Do you know anyone within your organization who could undertake this role? Ask your manager and colleagues if they have any recommendations.

Clinical supervision

In the UK, clinical supervision for nurses was introduced in the late 1980s. Since then it has become an integral part of clinical governance and quality assurance in the public health system (Mills et al. 2005). Skills for Care (2007: 4) define 'supervision' as 'an accountable process which supports, assures and develops the knowledge skills and values of an individual group or team'.

Reflection is often a way to recognize different approaches or ways of doing things leading to personal or team development, and Chapter 6 explores this in depth.

Supervision is usually between two individuals and is often seen by organizations as a way to promote personal and professional development in their staff (Jasper 2006). There are multiple types of supervision which can overlap, but the most common are managerial, professional, and clinical. These characteristics are shown in Table 8.2.

Midwifery have a separate type of supervision, with Supervisors of Midwives, defined by the NMC as experienced midwives who have had additional training and education to enable them to help midwives provide the best quality midwifery care (NMC 2016b). However, this role is currently being reviewed, and models to replace this are being evaluated. If you are a registered midwife or

Table 8.2 Types of clinical supervision

Managerial supervision	Carried out by a supervisor with the focus on: • Reviewing job performance. • Identifying strengths and weaknesses to plan further education and development needs. • Setting priorities and objectives to meet organizational and service needs.
Professional supervision	This refers to supervision which is carried out by another staff member from the same profession or group. Given this, professional aspects can be addressed such as: • Maintaining professional standards. • Planning and reviewing professional training. • Maintaining, or having a discussion around, professional codes of conduct within practice.
Clinical supervision	This tends to be a discussion in relation to practice. It can cover: • Reflection and review of practice within the clinical setting. • Focused discussion of practice, including specific cases, patients, episodes or events. • Action planning for the future to allow development or review of practice.

you work within a midwifery environment, look on the NMC website for the most up-to-date information. If you are a registered midwife you should consider how this evolving role may be able to help you with revalidation now and in the future. For example, you may choose your supervisor to be your reflective discussion partner. Another work-based relationship that can assist is that of critical companionship, and this is discussed next.

Critical companionship

Titchen (2000) describes this as a journey where an experienced facilitator accompanies another on an 'experiential learning journey' using methods of 'high challenge' and 'high support' in a trusting relationship. This may take the format of observing practice, or be in relation to written work. The basis of the relationship is improvement through feedback that encourages development, and as such it is perceived as fair and honest. If you have a critical companion you may wish to consider asking them to be your reflective discussion partner.

Time Out

Consider the benefits of critical companionship. Do you have a colleague in mind who could undertake this role?

They can be from another profession, but if they are not a registered nurse or midwife then remember they can't be your reflective discussion partner for revalidation purposes.

Another type of support you may already have access to is action learning. Often this is part of a course or as part of your ongoing professional development you may join an action learning set.

Action learning

Action learning builds on the relationship between reflection and action where understanding actions and looking for possible ways to solve problems is undertaken (McGill and Brockbank 2004). This is usually performed by formulation of a 'set' of people and initially a facilitator to guide the session. A presenter explains an issue they have, and the set actively listen to the issue and, at this point, ask questions for clarification only. Following this the set will question more deeply, often with 'what, who, why, when, can I just understand?', and cumulating with what they want to do – thus fulfilling the objective of helping the presenter come to their own solution. The questions are to be open and are definitely not to give advice or personal options to the presenter. This focus leads them to a plan of action to address concerns which fits with their way of working and thinking. Often the next time the set meets they will feed back on how this has gone.

Pause for Thought

Consider how you can use feedback from action learning as part of your revalidation evidence. This could be used as CPD, a reflective account, or as an example of practice-related feedback.

You may have other informal opportunities within your area, and shadowing is an example of this.

Shadowing

Shadowing is an opportunity to spend time with another professional observing them in action, which can improve your understanding of other areas of practice and job roles. It is important to have a clear idea of the outcomes that you wish to achieve and it is good to have this in mind when planning your shadowing visit. You would usually shadow an individual, but you could also shadow a meeting or event, and this would also give you the opportunity to further develop your professional network. Despite this being a learning experience for you, do not forget that you will also have experiences and knowledge that may be of direct benefit to the person you are shadowing – even chief executives like to know what is going on at a different level within their organization.

Shadowing may be something that you did some time ago, perhaps as a student, but have not revisited. However, key benefits may include:

- Giving you the opportunity to understand how another job role or department operates, with first-hand experience leading to an improved knowledge base.
- Setting up future networking opportunities (see next section).
- Providing career direction as the shadowing experience may confirm you wish to pursue a role in that speciality or area.
- Improving communication for both sides – this will occur naturally through both setting up the shadowing experience, during it, and subsequent interaction.
- Being able to learn and reflect from others (both parties may experience this).
- Giving better strategic or political awareness by exposing you to a higher level within the organization, and a subsequent understanding of how this influences key decisions and practice.
- Improving your influencing skills and negotiating skills by negotiating the experience, and influencing how it happens.

Be aware that there may be instances where shadowing in a particular meeting or situation is not possible due to confidentiality or health and safety. Where this is the case, you may have to alter your learning objectives or arrange another date – e.g. a case conference in child protection may have very limited space for health professionals and an additional member of staff would not be acceptable.

Pause for Thought

Before you arrange a shadowing opportunity, consider if you can use this experience for your revalidation evidence.

Could you use this experience as CPD or an opportunity to seek feedback?

After shadowing, ensure that you record and reflect on your learning as this can be utilized for many parts of your revalidation evidence. For example, this might be CPD, practice-related feedback, and you may choose to do a written reflection on how you have changed your practice.

If you are looking to develop your professional practice then networking is a key skill you want to possess.

Networking

When considering networking we usually think of the people around us in our working or personal life with a common interest or experience. You may find the concept of networking daunting, and Box 8.1 gives some key tips to getting started.

Box 8.1: Tips to help when networking

- Before you start it may be useful to think who you want to speak to and why – e.g. has that person got the job that you aspire to? Do you admire their skills?

- Be yourself; there is no point in not being honest and genuine and this potentially could prevent a good rapport developing with the individual.
- As with all communication, try not to dominate – both ask questions, listen and use open body language with a smile! Consider 'ice breakers' such as 'Do you work within this town or city? Which speciality or field of practice do you work in?'
- Think of individuals you know in the first instance before approaching either people you do not know, or very senior staff. Can they introduce you to them?
- Do you have a friend in business who is good at this? Why not ask them about their experiences as it may assist you.
- Include personal and professional interests – the ward manager who takes his child to the same football club as yours shows a common interest.
- Where you do not have a common interest, on meeting try and find one so the conversation flows easily. Be prepared to share some details about yourself – these do not need to be personal. Remember to keep the conversation as professional as possible.
- Be proactive! If you are thinking of approaching someone you don't know, or a more senior member of staff, consider what you are going to say carefully. If you act in a professional manner the worst that can happen is a short conversation that does not develop further.
- Consider opportunities to network at formal events – e.g. conferences, study days etc.
- Remember to have a purpose if you develop the relationship as quality is more important than quantity!!
- If you agree to follow up with an email or telephone call, ensure that you do.
- Ask yourself what you want to achieve? Are you looking for support with revalidation generally, or are you seeking a reflective discussion partner or confirmer?

Gibson et al. (2014) report that an agreed definition within the literature regarding networking is problematic, but common themes include those shown in Table 8.3.

Table 8.3 Common themes within networking (adapted from Gibson et al. 2014)

Area	Relevance to nursing practice
Networks (both internal and external) are useful to support career information and development.	These may include individuals from other countries or areas, or different professional groups, and will offer a wider view or give examples of innovation and developments which can assist you in your career aspirations.
Networking involves a behavioural response which enables and develops interpersonal skills.	This may include formation of friendships or mutual 'liking' through joint identification of goals or mutual benefits. This could also include information exchange.
Networking involves making connections with individuals who are perceived to be of benefit to your job role but are not immediate bosses or subordinates.	Making professional connections with senior managers from another hospital or speciality with a view to learning from them to improve job performance.
Individuals may identify and seek contact with those who they perceive to have tools to develop their work or career.	This suggests individuals with more knowledge or seniority than you. This could be through an internal contact, e.g. senior management engagement, or an external one, e.g. at a national conference.

Time Out

List or draw (see below) individuals that you network with both within your professional and personal life. If you want, you can further analyse what aspect(s) they fulfil utilizing Table 8.1 – in some cases you may not have realized that this was the case!

You may have detailed people you network with in a variety of ways that may include communicating:

- Face-to-face.
- Telephone conversations.
- Video conferencing.
- Email.

- Twitter.
- Facebook.
- Instant messaging.
- Community of practice.
- Journal clubs.
- Groups online e.g. Research Gate, LinkedIn etc.
- Through multidisciplinary learning activities.
- Other methods.

It is useful to frequently revisit the individuals within your network and what your desired outcome is so that you can achieve the best results. Some people are very good at networking, and this can be due to good interpersonal and communication skills ensuring both sides engage in the process. Ultimately, networks can help us cope with stress, develop ideas, and foster both our personal and professional development.

Your network can be used to help support you with revalidation. For example, your colleagues may be able to support you with the actual revalidation process, especially those that have already completed it. Alternatively your family may be able to support you with things like IT where you want to develop the skills to create an electronic portfolio. Where you work as a sole practitioner you may need to expand your network to include registrants who can fulfil the roles of reflective discussion partner and/or confirmer, if appropriate. A key part of networking is the ability to influence others.

Influencing others

Self-awareness is covered in the reflection chapter (Chapter 6), but another aspect to consider when engaging in a supportive relationship is what you can influence as an individual. Stephen Covey (2004) talks about individuals being either proactive or reactive, and within this how we deal with the areas in our life we can and cannot influence. He talks about two circles, one of concern and one of influence, and they sit within each other (see Figure 8.1). The circle of concern includes things like the NMC, your organization, pay bands, annual leave etc., whereas the circle of influence are things we can direct, which includes

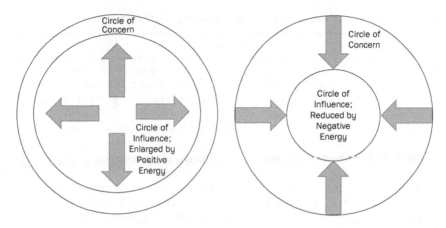

Figure 8.1 Circle of concern and circle of influence (adapted from Covey 2004)

things we have actual direct control over such as what education you decide to undertake, your attitude to work, what area of practice you want to work in, etc.

Covey (2004) believes that proactive people focus on the circle of influence where they can make changes and their energy is positive and increases in capacity, which in turn actively encourages the circle of influence to increase. Conversely, reactive people focus on the circle of concern which often involves the blaming of others and is correlated with negative energy and reduced activity in areas they can influence, thus causing their circle of influence to be reduced. A comparison of proactive and reactive characteristics adapted from Covey's model is shown in Table 8.4.

Time Out

Look at the characteristics of each list above. Which characteristics do you think most accurately describes you? Are you mainly proactive or reactive?

If you identified yourself as proactive you are spending time on things that you can change, which then expands the circle of influence. If you were more reactive you may worry about areas you

Table 8.4 A comparison of proactive and reactive characteristics

Proactive	Reactive
• Aware of your individual responsibilities and responses to events. • Very clear about your personal values and that your choices are made by you. • You do not blame or criticize others in order to make excuses for yourself. • Since you take ownership for your actions you control where you are going actively. • You tend to gravitate to the circle of influence as it is here that you can change things. You will still have a circle of concern, and Covey (2004) states that this will be at least as big as the circle of influence as you accept the ability of utilizing your influence effectively.	• You let external events and people influence how you behave and feel. This may include your mood and attitude. • You believe that how you 'are' is due to environmental or social aspects of life, and not determined by you as an individual. • You often make excuses or blame others for actions or events that occur. • You tend to operate within the circle of concern, focusing on the action of others leading, in some cases, to feelings of victimization. This causes their circle of influence to shrink – e.g. I am not successful in being sent on that course as my manager is blocking me.

Adapted from Covey (2004)

cannot change or effect, and the circle of influence may diminish. In relation to accessing education, consider the following case study:

Case study 1

Nurse Maria Sanchez wishes to undertake a one-day course in mindfulness. She has been waiting for her manager to put her forward for this and has become very frustrated with the situation. In addition, she has noticed that she has inadvertently blamed the manager for this not happening and noted that she perceives that others have had educational opportunities before her. Her happiness at both work and home have started to be affected by her attitude and mood.

If she were to become more proactive and focus on working within her circle of influence she might see more positive outcomes. This may involve getting a learning contract or agreement from her manager in order to plan when this will occur, and not 'wait' for others to influence this change for her. This would have the advantage of Nurse Maria Sanchez achieving her educational goal, and her happiness and well-being will also improve (and, in turn, this would increase her circle of influence).

Covey (2004) acknowledges that, at times, life can seem unfair and challenging, but the key is how you choose to deal with it, and your attitude can have a major effect. He describes a simple exercise which can have a big effect on your life and which will include planning your learning. Within your circle of influence, he suggests making small commitments (but ensuring you undertake them), being less judgemental or making excuses, and being active in problem-solving rather than contributing to the problem. Where you make mistakes (we all do), admit them, correct them, and learn from them – this may result in you making changes to yourself or your practice. In relation to others he suggests being compassionate and understanding to reduce blame and accept weaknesses. Individuals who do this expand their freedom and, in return, become effective in controlling their happiness and circumstances. Why not give it a try – and remember to record your reflections, if appropriate, as evidence for revalidation.

Summary

This chapter has explored the range of supportive relationships you can develop within your practice. Some of these roles you may already be familiar with, and some less so. By exploring and developing some of these supportive relationships you may be able to find support throughout your revalidation journey. You may wish to use what you have learned about influencing others or developing a network to expand the number of supportive relationships you have access to. It is a good idea to discuss some of these opportunities with your manager at the same time as your annual appraisal as you will be thinking about and planning your personal development at this time. If you work in isolation you may need to consider if you need to develop supportive relationships to ensure you have access to a reflective discussion partner and/or a confirmer if required (see the NMC website for the most up-to-date information on selecting a reflective discussion partner and/or confirmer). Overall, developing supportive relationships within your practice will provide opportunities for you to gain practice-related feedback, reflect on your practice, and undertake further continuing professional development.

Key points

- There are a range of supportive relationships you can access.
- These can be formal, informal, or regulatory in nature.
- These relationships can not only support you to gain confidence with the revalidation process but can also help you provide evidence to meet the required standards.
- Establishing a network can help you access support when needed.

Confirmation and the role of the confirmer

Introduction

Every registrant must be confirmed via a third party that they have met the NMC revalidation requirements (NMC 2015e). This person is chosen by the registrant and is known as the 'confirmer'. The confirmer has the responsibility of confirming the registrant has met the requirements of revalidation, and this role has been clearly defined by the NMC. The confirmer is the *only* person who can sign to confirm the revalidation requirements have been met. The confirmer is not being asked to verify the health and character or the professional indemnity insurance requirements. These are self-declarations made as part of the online renewal of registration application process. The confirmer is being asked to be honest and truthful when confirming a registrant, and should act with the best of their knowledge and belief. They do not have to be a registered nurse or midwife (NMC 2015f).

This chapter will outline the role of the confirmer and what confirmation means from a practical perspective. We will approach this role from both perspectives – that of the registrant who is providing evidence for revalidation, and the confirmer who is responsible for checking the revalidation requirements have been met.

Learning objectives

By the end of this chapter you will be able to:

- Explain the role of the confirmer.
- Describe the requirements for confirmation.

- Reflect and prepare for the confirmation discussion for your revalidation.

Revalidation Requirements Reminder

450 practice hours
35 hours of CPD
Five pieces of practice-related feedback
Five reflective accounts
Reflective discussion
Confirmation
Declaration of good health and character
Declaration of professional indemnity insurance.

(NMC 2015e)

Confirmation should only take place once the registrant has completed all of the requirements for revalidation, including their reflective discussion. However, if your confirmer is a registered nurse or midwife then this reflective discussion can take place at the same time as confirmation.

Current NMC revalidation requirements

The NMC (NMC 2015e: 28) states that:

'You [will] have demonstrated to an appropriate confirmer that you have complied with the revalidation requirements.'

Always refer to the NMC website for the most up-to-date revalidation guidance.

Choosing a confirmer

The NMC have defined a confirmer as an appropriate person, selected by the registrant, who will 'confirm' they have met the requirements for revalidation (NMC 2015f). This person is usually a line manager – however, some registrants may not have a line manager, for example if they are self-employed. These registrants will have to seek out an appropriate person, preferably another registrant, within their wider professional network (see Chapter 8). The purpose of confirmation is to provide assurance that a third party has checked the registrant has met the requirements for revalidation.

An appropriate confirmer could be:

- Line manager (they do not have to be a registrant).
- NMC registrant (either a registered nurse or registered midwife with effective registration – e.g. they cannot be retired, no longer registered, suspended or removed from the register at the time of confirmation).
- Other healthcare registered professional (e.g. a doctor, pharmacist).
- Other social care registered professional (e.g. a social worker, care home manager).

See the NMC website for a list of suitable confirmers.

Multiple roles

Some registrants will have multiple roles and multiple employers – for example, they may have a substantive post as a health visitor and work part-time as a nurse on the staff bank.

Others may be on more than one part of the register – for example, they are a registered nurse and a registered midwife. Each registrant will only need to have one confirmation meeting no matter how many roles they have or how many parts of the register they are on. In these situations, it is for the registrant to decide who their confirmer should be; however, the NMC recommend that these registrants select a confirmer from the role they practise most frequently in. This is because the confirmer will be most familiar with the registrant's practice, which should make the confirmation discussion more meaningful for both parties. Although this level of familiarity is desirable, it is not essential (NMC 2015f).

No line manager

For those registrants who do not have access to a line manager it is suggested by the NMC (2015e) that the first option should be to try and approach another NMC registrant to undertake the role of confirmer. If this is not possible, then they should approach either a registered healthcare professional or a registered social care professional who has worked with them. This person does not have to be familiar with your practice, but they must be familiar with the most up-to-date NMC revalidation guidance (NMC 2015e) and have read the most up-to-date NMC confirmer guidance (NMC 2015f). Your confirmer does not have to be a higher band or grade than you; they may be in a position either more junior or more senior to you – it is for you to decide who would be most suited to this role. However, you should be aware of your professional responsibilities when selecting your confirmer and you should be aware of any conflicts of interest. For example, they should not be a friend or family member, and you should try to avoid someone you are commercially linked to (NMC 2015e).

Time Out

Find out when you are due to revalidate by registering with NMC Online (see Chapter 2 and the NMC website).

Find out who your confirmer is likely to be. If they are a registrant you must check if they will also be your reflective discussion partner.

Do you foresee any conflicts of interest?

Start considering your actions in relation to this now!

Some nurses or midwives who work within a bank, agency or independent setting may find it challenging to find a confirmer. If you cannot find a confirmer and have explored all of the options set out above, then you should contact the NMC for advice. It is important that you make decisions regarding your confirmer as soon as possible. Do not leave this until you are just about to renew your registration! Identify your confirmer or any issues in doing this early, and approach your confirmer well in advance.

Pause for Thought

Remember: you can have your confirmation discussion at any point in the 12 months leading up to your revalidation date.

Further on in this chapter we will give a checklist for registrants to consider when preparing for their confirmation, and will look at the confirmation discussion in more detail. First though, we will consider the support that is expected to be given by an employer.

Employer responsibilities

Employers will be expected to support registrants to achieve the requirements for their re-registration. The NMC have produced an employer guide which sets out the expectations for revalidation support for those who employ registrants (NMC 2015g). This includes providing support for them to meet the revalidation requirements. It is the individual registrant's responsibility to maintain their registration, and there is no onus upon the employer to do this on behalf of the registrant. They are not required to support paid time out of practice to allow revalidation requirements to be met – for example, for continuing professional development to take place (NMC 2015g). However, it is in the best interests of the registrant and the employer to develop their staff. This leads to improved morale and job satisfaction, and also improves the quality of care being delivered (Borrill et al. 2002).

As revalidation is a new system, there may be anxieties about how this will work in practice. It is important to have clear communication within any organization employing nurses or midwives in relation to this as early as possible. Anxiety can be reduced by ensuring any staff involved in revalidation from a confirmer or registrant perspective have access to the facts and understand the requirements for revalidation. It is important to check the NMC website regularly for any changes and updates as an employer, confirmer, or as a registrant.

The revalidation model was developed with a range of practice settings in mind, so should be workable regardless of your employment model. If you employ registrants, the NMC employer guidance (NMC 2015g) sets out the minimum support expected in relation to four key areas.

The NMC have suggested employers should focus on these areas of support for registrants:

1   Awareness and culture – it is reasonable to expect employers to raise awareness of revalidation among registrants and, where possible, communicate the NMC's revalidation requirements.

2   Capacity and capability of resources – ensuring the organiza-
    tion supports registrants by allowing time and opportunity for
    reflective and confirmation discussions.
3   Systems and processes – these should ensure all registrants can
    revalidate by supporting access to IT equipment and encourag-
    ing them to register with NMC Online.
4   Guidance, tools and support – it is important to signpost regis-
    trants to the resources, tools and guidance on the NMC website.

While you are expected to be supportive, as an employer you must
emphasize that the responsibility for meeting the revalidation
requirements rests with the individual registrant (NMC 2015e).

Pause for Thought

If a registrant is undergoing a local disciplinary procedure or an NMC
fitness to practise investigation, this does not stop them from seeking
and obtaining confirmation, providing they meet the necessary requirements and they have not been suspended or struck off from the NMC
register.

(NMC 2015f)

Supporting registrants with revalidation

There may be some anxiety or uncertainty around whether nurses
and midwives working in non-clinical roles are able to revalidate.
You may be asked to confirm these registrants, so it is important that
you are clear what your role is.

The confirmer has to be satisfied that the registrant has practised
the minimum number of hours required for registration. This can be
in a paid clinical role, a voluntary role, or a non-clinical role such as
education or policy development. It is worth noting that the NMC
states that any hours obtained as a healthcare assistant or support
worker cannot be counted as practice hours as a registered nurse or
midwife (NMC 2015e). Any registrant in a non-nursing post must be
able to provide evidence that they have been practising using their

nursing knowledge, skills and experience. Evidence may consist of anything which proves the hours they have worked and used their nursing knowledge, skills and experience; this may include payslips, job descriptions or an employment contract which describes their role and responsibilities. They may present their evidence on the appropriate NMC template, which is likely to include a description of their practice setting, dates of practice, scope of practice, a description of the work undertaken and number of hours. This form isn't mandatory at this time, but is very helpful because it sets out the NMC's revalidation requirements. It is worth noting that these practice hours are unchanged from the original PREP requirements (NMC 2011).

Continuing professional development (CPD)

Continuing professional development is something which all registrants have been required to do since PREP began (NMC 2011). However, the participatory learning hours are a new requirement for revalidation. As an employer you can support nurses and midwives to access participatory learning and work-based learning. This may be as simple as signposting registrants to activities or events which may help them meet the revalidation requirements. This may form part of the personal development planning and appraisal process. You may also encourage registrants to log their CPD using the most up-to-date templates and tools from the NMC website (see Chapter 4 for more details on meeting the CPD requirements).

Feedback

Registrants may be unsure about where they can source feedback, and it is useful if you can support this as an employer or as a confirmer. Feedback can be positive or constructive, and you can support registrants in a number of ways, either by giving them feedback directly or by encouraging others to give feedback as part of a learning culture within practice. You may also have a role in encouraging registrants to seek feedback by signposting them to opportunities that may exist. These may include looking at audit reports or compliments or complaints received. Feedback should be integral to practice, and not something the registrant should have to seek out (NMC 2015e).

Reflective accounts

These must be five written accounts based on their CPD and/or practice-related feedback and/or an event or experience in practice, and how this relates to the Code (NMC 2015a). Supporting reflective discussions as part of team meetings can be helpful, as can building reflective practice into appraisal or PDP discussions.

Preparing for confirmation

Confirmers and registrants must read the most up-to-date NMC Confirmer Guide (NMC 2015f) and NMC Revalidation Guide (NMC 2015e), which are available from NMC website, prior to the confirmation meeting.

Pause for Thought

Your renewal expiry will be the end of the month, but your revalidation date will be the first of the month; this is when you should have made your online declaration through 'NMC Online' to guarantee your re-registration.

This change is very important because the implications of not meeting the portal deadline may result in the registrant not being registered with the NMC; therefore they will be unable to practise until reinstated.

Registrant checklist

You are ready to arrange your confirmer meeting when:

- ✓ You have identified your confirmer.
- ✓ You have spoken with your confirmer and agreed that they will undertake that role.
- ✓ You have collated all of your evidence.
- ✓ You have had your reflective discussion with another registrant (unless you are going to have this as part of your confirmation meeting).
- ✓ You have less than 12 months until you are due to revalidate.

Confirmation meeting

When you are preparing for your confirmation meeting and collecting all of your evidence, you should review your practice and consider how you can demonstrate that you are continuing to meet the principles and values set out in the Code (NMC 2015a). You should review all of the information against the most up-to-date NMC revalidation guidance to ensure you have met the minimum requirements. This will also help to refresh your memory as some of the evidence you have obtained may be up to 3 years old, and reviewing your evidence will also help you to answer any questions or queries your confirmer may have. When collating your revalidation information, make sure you store this in a format that will be easy for your confirmer to access and read. You may hold your evidence electronically or in paper format, ensuring you are familiar with data protection laws (see Chapter 10). Your confirmer may ask for this evidence to be sent to them prior to the confirmation meeting.

The confirmation meeting can take place at any point in the final 12 months before your revalidation date, or earlier, but only in exceptional circumstances (you should contact the NMC for advice). You should mutually agree the date, time and place, ensuring there will be no interruptions. You should also ensure you bring your evidence and can get access to your online portfolio, if you have one.

Ensure enough time is allowed for a full discussion to take place. The NMC have not defined how long this should take. It is worth clarifying expectations with your confirmer in advance as to how long you should allow. It is likely to take around an hour. The time this is likely to take will depend on how familiar your confirmer is with your practice and the evidence you have provided. This meeting should be held face-to-face, preferably in person, but if this is not possible then video conference facilities can be used.

Confirmation meeting

Make sure you have the most up-to-date mandatory NMC confirmation template in front of you, which can be downloaded from the NMC website. It might be easier if you both have a copy to look at, but only one copy is required to be completed to meet the revalidation requirements. If you are likely to be confirming a number of registrants, or have had a confirmation meeting early in the 12 months prior to the revalidation date of the registrant, it is worth keeping accurate records of when you had the confirmation meeting. This is for your own records because the NMC may want to verify that the meeting took place. Ensuring you meet data protection laws is important when storing personal information about a registrant (see Chapter 10).

If evidence is sent in advance of the meeting and is insufficient then this must be addressed at the time rather than waiting until the confirmation meeting takes place unless you feel some points just require some further explanation.

The confirmation process does not assess quality of evidence; that is the registrant's responsibility (NMC 2015f). However, you may feel as a confirmer that you can give some constructive feedback on the quality and scope of evidence you see, but this should not prevent confirmation from taking place. This may be helpful for the registrant's ongoing personal and professional development, and completing confirmation at the same time as their appraisal supports this process.

Pause for Thought

Key questions for confirmers:

Has the registrant met the minimum requirements?
If not, why have these not been met?
What needs to be done?
When does this need to be completed?
What support can you offer?

The confirmation discussion

You should be prepared to discuss each aspect of the requirements with your confirmer as detailed in Table 9.1.

Table 9.1 Revalidation requirements

Revalidation requirement	Standard	Evidence
450 practice hours	The registrant should be able to provide evidence of their practice hours, if required.	Payslips, timesheets or employment contracts are a good source of evidence of hours worked. If you are very familiar with the registrant's practice you may not require to see written evidence of practice hours.
35 hours of CPD (including 20 participatory learning hours)	The registrant must be able to produce evidence detailing a minimum of 35 hours CPD, of which 20 hours *must* be participatory.	These records must contain: • The CPD method. • A description of the topic and how it related to their practice. • The dates on which the activity was undertaken. • The number of hours (including the number of participatory hours). • Identification of the part of the Code most relevant to the activity. • Evidence that they undertook the CPD activity – this may include certificates, reflections, learning outcomes, letters, programmes or presentations. Any form can be used to record this information, but it is desirable to use the most up-to-date NMC templates available from the NMC website.
Five pieces of practice-related feedback	The registrant must be able to describe the feedback they have received.	Evidence can be written or oral, include feedback through involvement in incidents or complaints, and informal or formal comments from patients, carers, colleagues.

(Continued)

Table 9.1 (Continued)

Revalidation requirement	Standard	Evidence
	Feedback should be considered in its broadest context, and does not need to be sought formally. It is important that the registrant has received and recognized this feedback.	In addition, this can include appraisal or feedback from managers, as well as audit reports and findings from incident reviews.
Five written reflections	The registrant must be able to provide written records of reflection.	Evidence will be presented on the mandatory NMC approved form. The reflections should explain what the registrant has learned from the CPD Activity and/or practice-related feedback and/or an event or experience in their practice, how they have changed or improved their work as a result, and how this is relevant to the Code (NMC 2015a).
Reflective discussion	The registrant will provide evidence of the reflective discussion. If the confirmer is an NMC registrant, they can undertake this discussion at the same time as confirmation. However, if they are NOT an NMC registrant, the registrant revalidating will have to have a separate discussion with an NMC registrant prior to confirmation.	Evidence will be presented on the mandatory NMC approved form. This will provide a written record of the reflective discussion, signed by the registrant and their reflective discussion partner.
Confirmation	All of the evidence above must satisfy the confirmer that the standard has been reached.	This will be recorded on the mandatory NMC approved form, signed and dated by you as the confirmer.

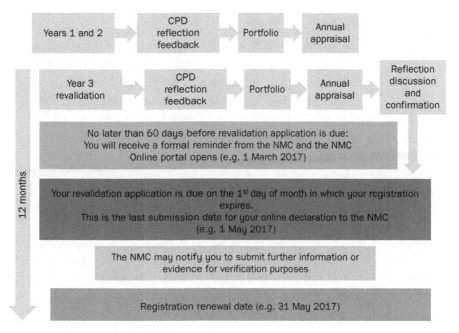

Figure 9.1 Flowchart of the revalidation process

Figure 9.1 shows an overview of the revalidation process, which may be useful in reviewing where you are in your revalidation journey.

Raising concerns

Confirmers are expected to act in good faith and with honesty. They are being asked to consider whether the nurse or midwife has met the requirements for revalidation, based on the evidence supplied and the discussions that have taken place (NMC 2015f). However, if there has been any breach of the Code (NMC 2015a) during the revalidation process this can lead to a separate fitness-to-practise investigation. This applies to the registrant and the confirmer if they are registered with the NMC or another regulator.

Scenario 1

'What if I am a confirmer or reflective partner and I have concerns about the evidence I see?'

Points to consider:

If you are doing either a reflective conversation or confirmation discussion and view any evidence which calls into question the registrant's fitness to practise, this is a separate issue. This must be discussed with the registrant and escalated through the appropriate employer channels and processes in the first instance.

If the registrant is independently employed, with no line manager, then a direct referral to the NMC may be appropriate. Providing the registrant has met the requirements for revalidation they must be confirmed as their registration will lapse without this. A registrant may lapse if they have failed to meet the requirements, but they should be given an opportunity to rectify this. The only organization who can remove a registrant from the register is the NMC. Without current registration the NMC would be unable to investigate a registrant's fitness to practise, which would not be in the public interest. Revalidation is not a way of removing nurses who are poorly performing from the register.

If you have any queries you should contact the NMC for advice.

Confirmation concerns

Revalidation is not about assessing the quality of the evidence, although it is important that your confirmer understands that the evidence needs to meet the requirements. The confirmer is not expected to seek third-party assurance of the declaration or evidence produced by the registrant.

Scenario 2

What if you do not agree with your confirmer or what if your evidence doesn't satisfy your confirmer?

Points to consider:

You must allow time to resubmit your evidence to your confirmer and to have an additional confirmation discussion. If you are told your evidence is insufficient then ensure you are clear what is missing or how you can meet the requirements. You should understand what you need to complete, and by when. It's important to clarify what you need to do to meet the standards required. If you cannot resolve this issue and your confirmer remains concerned it is important that you involve a third party at this stage. If you feel you have met the requirements you should be able to consult with your employer or professional lead within your organization and raise any concerns about the confirmation process and your confirmer.

If you have any queries you should contact the NMC for advice.

Confirmation should be a supportive process where you have an opportunity to demonstrate you are fit *for* practice as a registrant. This is not to be confused with the regulatory fitness *to* practise processes. The confirmer or employer should support this. If the registrant is unable to revalidate they will lapse from the NMC register and have to apply for re-entry. The NMC have specific guidance on the process which has to be followed if a registrant fails to submit a revalidation application in time, and more details of this can be found on the NMC website. Clearly, if a registrant is unable to revalidate and their registration lapses, this has significant implications for the registrant and the employer. This may in turn lead to a separate internal investigation as to the reasons for their registration lapsing.

Top Tips

Support

It is important if you are going through revalidation for the first time or are confirming someone for the first time that you seek peer support. Have any of your colleagues already been through the process? Did you ask them for any top tips? Is there anything that would support you? Can you shadow a more experienced confirmer, or would they support you if you are unsure? (See Chapter 8.)

Reflection

After you have completed confirmation, either as a registrant or as a confirmer, it is important to reflect on the process. You could ask yourself three simple questions: What went well? What didn't go so well? What would I do differently next time? (For more detailed models of reflection, see Chapter 6.)

Time

Allow enough time for the meeting to be a quality discussion – this shouldn't be rushed!

Encourage the registrant to allow enough time for the confirmation meeting before the final guaranteed submission date of the first of the month of their re-registration date.

Progress

As a registrant, reflect on your own progress and make a plan of what you need to complete before you have your confirmation discussion.

As a confirmer, you should monitor progress at every annual appraisal, set goals, and benchmark against the NMC Revalidation Guidance (NMC 2015e) to support the registrant to meet the revalidation standards.

Case study: Confirmer

Role: Regional manager of a care home.

Situation: You have been asked to confirm two care home managers in your region over the next few months, but you are new in post so you don't know any of them particularly well.

Points to consider: You don't need to be familiar with their practice, but you do need to be clear about your role as confirmer. This includes your need to be clear about the process of revalidation and the need to understand what the registrant expects from the meeting. Consider how to facilitate two-way feedback, reflect on the process, and identify what you have learned and if you have any further learning needs.

If you have any queries you should contact the NMC for advice.

Case study: Registrant

Role: Chief executive of a charity within the independent sector.

Situation: You are not employed as a registered nurse, but have been using your nursing knowledge and skills within your practice.

You only see your line manager four times per year as this is a national charity and head office is not close to where you work geographically. Your line manager is not a registrant. You are due to revalidate in 18 months.

Points to consider: As you can have your confirmation discussion 12 months in advance you have already spoken to your confirmer and organized this for your next one-to-one meeting. You also plan to send your evidence electronically to your confirmer prior to your meeting to allow time for them to consider this and ask any questions. You have sought out another registrant to have a reflective discussion with prior to your confirmation meeting. They work as a registered nurse for the same charity.

If you have any queries you should contact the NMC for advice.

Concerns about your confirmer

If you find yourself in a situation where you are unhappy with your confirmer for any reason, this should be raised at the earliest opportunity. You should not wait until you are due to have your confirmation meeting to raise these concerns. The NMC strongly recommend you obtain confirmation from your line manager however you can choose to have a different person other than your line manager to confirm you. You should also be mindful of the Code (NMC 2015a) when selecting a confirmer, particularly the fundamental tenets which include the need to be open and honest, act with integrity, and above all, uphold the reputation of the profession.

Appraisal

The easiest way of confirming your practice is to integrate your confirmation discussion into your existing appraisal processes. Revalidation is not a single event at one point in time; it should be part of a three-yearly cycle of planning your evidence and checking your progress towards meeting the revalidation requirements. In the majority of cases your confirmer will be your line manager. This should be the same person who normally does your appraisal, and if you don't have a regular appraisal, revalidation may give you the opportunity to request one.

This will give you the opportunity to discuss your revalidation evidence with your line manager at least once a year. Ideally your line manager will conduct your appraisal and they will also be your confirmer; this prevents confirmation taking place in isolation (NMC 2015f). Any concerns about your evidence, or how you are meeting the revalidation requirements, can then be raised well in advance of the confirmation meeting.

Appraisal can complement the confirmation process and discussions on adherence to the NMC Code (NMC 2015a) and professionalism should form a core part of the appraisal process (NMC 2015e). Combining existing appraisal processes with revalidation can support the clear links between personal and professional development planning and safe and effective practice. This has benefits for both the individual registrant and their organization with training, development and workforce planning (Borrill et al. 2002).

> The appraisal process is part of a continual process of planning, monitoring, assessment and support to help staff develop their skills and be more effective in their role. The annual appraisal interview sits at the heart of the process. There is evidence both within the NHS and industry that an effective appraisal process increases the effectiveness of the organization.
>
> (Scottish Executive 2005: 69)

If you work for the NHS in the UK then your appraisal and PDP will be undertaken using the Knowledge and Skills Framework (KSF). The KSF process combines both appraisal and personal development so is more than just a process for appraising staff. The development review focuses on the individual's development, whereas appraisal focuses on the individual's performance in the job, including any specific personal objectives.

Even if your employer does not use KSF then they should still be carrying out appraisals to assist you with your ongoing personal and professional development; this is viewed as good employment practice. Depending on the organization you work for you may use this model or you may use something different; what is important is that it is an outcomes-based approach (RCN 2009). Each year you should be given the opportunity to have a discussion about your revalidation evidence and reflect on your practice, as part of your appraisal.

Here is an example of an alternative framework which describes an appraisal process with four key stages:

1   A self-assessment by the individual of strengths and development needs.
2   A structured discussion with the appraiser based on the self-assessment.
3   An agreed personal development plan which flows from the appraisal discussion.
4   Action to meet the learning needs identified in the personal development plan.

(Scottish Executive 2005: 69)

Appraisal should focus on how you do your job, rather than what you do for your job. It should build on the personal attributes you possess or may wish to develop (RCN 2009).

Some of the attributes you may wish to develop may include:

● Communication skills.
● Leadership skills.
● Problem-solving and decision-making skills.
● Time management skills.
● Autonomous working.
● Organizational skills.
● Staff management.
● Delegation of work.
● Teamworking.

(Scottish Executive 2005)

Time Out

The Code (NMC 2015a) promotes professionalism and is central to safe, effective nursing and midwifery practice.

Reread and reflect on The Code (NMC 2015a). When considering the attributes you wish to develop as part of your appraisal, can you link these to the sections of The Code?

Can you speak to your line manager about linking your annual appraisal to your confirmation meeting?

Summary

This chapter has explored the role of the confirmer and the requirements that are necessary to undertake the role – namely, to understand what the revalidation requirements are and how the process is undertaken. The key considerations have been explored to ensure the confirmation conversation is meaningful to both the registrant and the confirmer. Despite the NMC clearly defining revalidation as the key responsibility of the registrant (NMC 2015e) it is within the employer's best interest to support the process, and the four areas have been defined within the chapter. Issues which may arise either with the confirmer role or the process have been discussed using some case studies with the aim of explaining how some unusual circumstances can be overcome within practice. Finally, combining the confirmation discussion and the appraisal process are discussed to encourage readers to plan how to get the best out of their appraisal and professional development planning (PDP) – for more about this, see Chapter 4.

Key points

- Identify your confirmer, or if you will be expected to be a confirmer as soon as possible.
- Plan your confirmation meeting well in advance of your renewal or revalidation date.
- Be clear about the role of the confirmer, remembering that this is about checking the revalidation standards have been met; it is not about the quality of evidence produced.

10 Recording learning and portfolio development

This chapter will guide you through the process of portfolio development and support you to plan and record your learning. The ability to reflect on your learning and plan the next step in your development will help you progress your own learning as well as your career. It is important that you record your progress and achievements, including capturing the 'soft' outcomes and any unplanned learning. This chapter will also discuss gathering evidence to support the NMC revalidation requirements.

Learning objectives

By the end of this chapter you will be able to:

- Identify what you should record as evidence, in line with NMC revalidation requirements.
- Make a detailed plan to create a portfolio.
- Describe different ways of structuring portfolios, and use one of these to structure your own portfolio.
- Anonymize what you record in your portfolio.
- Summarize the main elements of a portfolio and how it can be used to inform your own development.

The NMC states that in relation to revalidation a portfolio is the preferred method of storing your evidence.

Current NMC revalidation requirements

The NMC (NMC 2015e:10) states that:

'We strongly recommend that you keep evidence that you have met the revalidation requirements in a portfolio. This does not necessarily need to be an e-portfolio.'

Always refer to the NMC website for the most up-to-date revalidation guidance.

What is a portfolio?

A professional portfolio is more than a collection of certificates and a CV, it should demonstrate a range of learning from a variety of different experiences. Scholes et al. (2004: 595) describe a portfolio as something that:

> 'Captures learning from experience, enables an assessor to measure student learning, acts as a tool for reflective thinking, illustrates critical analysis skills and evidence of self-directed learning and provides a collection of detailed evidence of a person's competence.'

The key to good portfolio development is the ability to recognize meaningful evidence of your achievements which best represents your professional development. You should, however, be selective when deciding on what evidence to include in your portfolio. By regularly reviewing your portfolio you can assess your progress towards your goals.

Critical thinking or critical reflection is an essential part of portfolio development, as it can provide evidence of the way you link theory to practice. In Chapter 6 there were several models of reflection which are discussed in detail that you can refer to and use to guide your portfolio development.

A portfolio can be used to store evidence of:

- Skills you have gained.
- Achievements at work.

- Qualifications.
- Feedback you have received.

(Clark 2010a)

Types of portfolio

Collating your evidence for revalidation in a portfolio is recommended by the NMC and you have two main choices of how to store and create your portfolio, either in paper or electronic format. There are many templates available to download if you choose to use a paper portfolio or you can create your own template using any of the structures described below. Electronic portfolios tend to have set templates within each system. There are both free and paid for providers of electronic portfolio or e-portfolios, as they are known; it really is your decision which you prefer, and for revalidation requirements either is suitable (NMC 2015e).

Time Out

Consider the benefits and limitations of a paper portfolio versus an electronic one. Consider your learning needs or learning style as described in Chapter 3 and what you want to use your portfolio for.

Paper

All you would require would be a ring binder and some dividers to begin your portfolio. This is probably the simplest one to have. The benefits of a paper portfolio are that they are easy to access, simple to update, and it is easy to add additional information; however, they are not easily accessible from any location. You have to physically carry your portfolio around, and it can become quite a large collection of documents.

Electronic

E-portfolios are easy to access from any location, and once you have all of your evidence uploaded they are simple to update, but you would require a computer or similar device plus an internet connection.

You don't have to carry hard copies around, but if you do want to store certificates then these would need to be scanned into the portfolio if they are in a paper format. However, you have to be careful not to get distracted by the use of technology.

You may already keep a professional portfolio. If so, you do not need to maintain a separate portfolio for revalidation – you can simply build on the existing portfolio and change it as required. Throughout your career what you need from a portfolio may change. Your portfolio needs to reflect this and can be used for many purposes.

You can use your portfolio throughout your career for:

- Revalidation.
- Preparation for your appraisal or development meeting.
- Continuing professional development (CPD).
- Personal development planning (PDP).
- Job or course application.
- Academic study or professional qualifications .
- Monitoring your practice – for example, if you are in a new role or are developing new skills.
- Career development or advancement.

(Pitts 2010)

Where to begin?

When planning your portfolio it is important you take a step-by-step approach to portfolio development (Timmins and Duffy 2011). By considering each of these steps you can ensure the best chance of success.

1 Decide to engage.
2 Commit.
3 Explore and consider different types of portfolios.
4 Identify the approach that works best for you, along with potential barriers to success.
5 Negotiate and discuss your thoughts and decisions so far with colleagues or a reflective friend or critical companion.
6 Plan your strategy based on realistic targets.
7 Implement your strategy in a disciplined manner.
8 Re-examine as you progress, periodically question and examine your personal attitudes and values.

9   Persist, as no matter what barriers fall in your way, providing evidence for revalidation is essential to maintain your registration with the NMC.

(Adapted from Timmins and Duffy 2011)

Time Out

Consider any barriers to developing your portfolio. Make a list of these and then plan how you will overcome these to ensure you stay on track with your portfolio development.

Some of the barriers you may have identified include lack of time, not knowing where to begin, and being unsure about how to structure your evidence. These can all be overcome by planning your portfolio and having a clear structure in mind (Clark 2010b).

Time Out

Consider the following key questions when planning your portfolio:

Purpose and audience

● Why are you developing a portfolio? Is it only for revalidation purposes?
● Who is your target audience? Do they have different requirements or can you use one portfolio to meet this and your revalidation needs?

Design of the portfolio

● Would you prefer paper-based or electronic?
● Do you want to use a portfolio provider/template or create your own?
● Is there a competence framework or a set of criteria that has to be used? Consider the revalidation guidance or the Code (NMC 2015a).

Contents of the portfolio

● What is your own or your organization's philosophy of nursing or midwifery?

What kind of material do you want to include:

- Written material – for example, reflective accounts, conference programmes.
- Visual material – for example, mind maps, PowerPoint presentations.
- Digital material – for example, pictures of flip charts, copies of articles you have written.

Recording and reflecting on your learning

You may want to include:

- A description of events, learning activities and/achievements.
- Evidence of your performance – for example, feedback, appraisal information.
- Choice of reflective model and your written reflective accounts.

(Forde et al. 2009)

Once you have decided on these you can consider the structure.

Structure

For revalidation purposes it is useful to collate your evidence in one place and it is worth considering how you may structure this. Deciding on the structure of your portfolio is usually best planned before you start your portfolio, either in advance of collating your evidence, or you can plan your structure at the start of your revalidation cycle. You may want to develop a mind map, which can be a useful tool for developing a structure for your portfolio (see Figure 10.1).

Pause for Thought

You must identify your revalidation cycle to know which dates you are collecting information from. For example, if you have renewed your registration on 31 August 2016 then you would be collecting evidence from 1 September 2016 until 31 August 2019 for your next revalidation cycle. You would have to be aware that your reflective discussion and confirmation would take place prior to the renewal date, so it is best to have your evidence completed approximately two to three months prior to when you are due to revalidate.

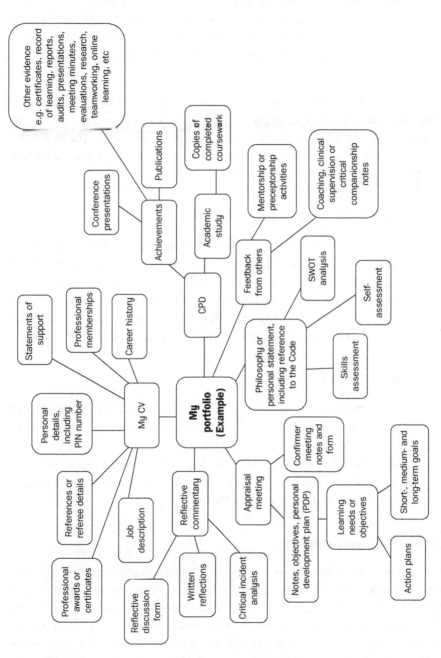

Figure 10.1 Example portfolio mind map

There is no correct way to structure your portfolio, so try not to feel overwhelmed when considering how to order everything. You want to be able to find evidence or information quickly and easily. You can have a separate section purely for your revalidation evidence, or you can thread this throughout the portfolio. There is no right or wrong way to do this.

There are many different ways of structuring your portfolio, but you may want to consider using a model. The main ones described by Timmins and Duffy (2011) are the 'Shopping Trolley', 'Toast Rack', 'Spinal Column' or 'Cake-mix' models – or, you can choose to use a combination of these or your own structure.

Shopping Trolley model

This is where you store your documents in any order or you may simply store your evidence chronologically. For example, you could simply store each piece of feedback, CPD activity, reflective account etc. as you complete them. This is not a meaningful way of developing your portfolio because there is no linkage between components, but it would enable you to store the evidence required for revalidation purposes.

Toast Rack model

This is a more structured way of organizing your evidence, using sections for each part of your evidence. For example, you could have a section for practice hours, reflective accounts, feedback etc. Again, this model would be suitable for revalidation purposes, but there is no linking element to this portfolio so it doesn't allow you to demonstrate the depth of your learning.

Spinal Column model

This is a way of using overarching themes to organize your evidence. For example, you could use the four overarching themes of the Code (NMC 2015a) and select the CPD, reflective accounts and feedback which you have aligned to these sections as evidence. Or you could use the four pillars of practice described in Chapter 4 which were 1) Clinical Practice, 2) Leadership and Management, 3) Facilitation of Learning, 4) Evidence, Research and Development (The Scottish Government 2008) and store a range of evidence under each heading.

This is a more meaningful way of storing your revalidation evidence because of the linkage between sections.

Cake-mix model

This is a more advanced way of building your portfolio and this type is often used for academic study. This portfolio involves linking all of your evidence together — this involves looking at your portfolio as a whole to identify what it tells you about your practice. Middleton (2011) suggests when considering this model it can help to ask yourself the following questions:

What? (the past) What have I collected about my work, learning, knowledge, skills and competence?

So what? (the present) What does this show about my practice and what I have learned?

Now what? (the future) In what direction do I want or need to go in the future?

This type of portfolio is more complex, but could be used for revalidation purposes – for example, the basis for this portfolio is likely to be a reflective commentary giving an overview of your learning and professional development across your three-year revalidation cycle. Within this reflective commentary you then make reference and add additional evidence within your portfolio, such as feedback, evidence of CPD, and reflective accounts. You are then able to add 'layers' and build your portfolio in this way, continuously reflecting and layering evidence demonstrating your development within your portfolio and which may explore a different aspect of the same event, or simply show your overall development. This model allows you to not only evidence your learning, but also your critical thinking.

What evidence is required?

To maintain your registration and meet the NMC revalidation requirements you must provide evidence of your practice hours, CPD, practice-related feedback, reflective accounts, reflective discussion and confirmation meetings (see Table 10.1). The NMC may also want to check some of this evidence for the purposes of verification (NMC 2015e). It is recommended you could store all of this evidence within your portfolio by downloading or printing off the most up-to-date NMC forms and templates. Check on the NMC website for the most up-to-date information on which templates and forms are mandatory and which are simply recommended.

Table 10.1 Requirements and evidence for revalidation

Requirement	Suggested evidence
450 practice hours	You should keep a record of your practice hours to demonstrate you have completed 450 hours across three years prior to revalidation. You can also complete the relevant NMC template.
Five pieces of practice-related feedback	You do not need to keep evidence of this, but it is recommended you keep a note of the content of any feedback you receive and how you have used this to reflect on your practice. Your confirmer will ask you about this. You can also complete the relevant NMC template.
Five reflective accounts	You must keep a record of at least five written reflective accounts on your CPD and/or practice-related feedback and/or an event in your practice over the three years. You will have to explain what you learned, how you changed or improved your work as a result, and how it is relevant to the Code (NMC 2015a). You must complete the relevant NMC template for each instance. Your reflective discussion partner and confirmer will want to see these.
35 hours continuing professional development	You must keep a record of any CPD relevant to your scope of practice, both participatory and non-participatory hours. You can complete the NMC template for each instance. Evidence that CPD has taken place may include certificates of attendance, records of learning, notes, signed letters etc. Your confirmer will want to see this.
Reflective discussion	You must keep a copy of the completed NMC form with details of the registrant with whom you have had the discussion. If this happens separately to confirmation, your confirmer will want to see this.
Confirmation from a third party	You will need to demonstrate to a third party that you have met the revalidation requirements. You must keep a copy of the completed relevant NMC form.
Professional indemnity	You will need to have evidence of your professional indemnity cover. If you work for the NHS this is part of your contract of employment, but if you work for a private or independent organization then this should be sourced and a copy kept. Your confirmer does not need to see this but you will need to declare to the NMC that you have this cover.
Health and character	You will make a self-declaration of this. No independent evidence is required.

Pause for Thought

Throughout your evidence, please ensure individuals cannot be identified and all information recorded is anonymized (see section on confidentiality later in this chapter).

Scoping existing portfolio evidence

You may already have a portfolio which you have had throughout your career. This might have been for another purpose such as appraisal or for further study. You may be able to use some of this evidence if it meets the requirements for revalidation. You can scope what you have by using the following questions, and then you should make a list of the evidence you still need to collect.

- Do I have any reflective accounts or reflective statements?
- Do I have any pieces of feedback from others relating to my practice as an individual or as a team?
- Do I have a log of the CPD I have undertaken?
- Do I have evidence that I have undertaken this CPD?

Once you have collated your portfolio it is for you to select the most important or pertinent evidence to meet the revalidation requirements. You may wish to discuss your portfolio evidence regularly during your annual appraisal as this will allow you time to collect any additional information if required. You may also wish to discuss this with your confirmer or with a peer prior to your reflective discussion and/or confirmation. This evidence must meet the current revalidation standards, therefore it is important that you check the NMC for the most up-to-date templates and guidance.

Examples of types of evidence

The types of evidence you may want to include in your portfolio may include:

Self-assessment.
Action plans.

CPD plans.
Learning logs.
Certificates.
Reflective accounts.
Examples of work which evidence skills development.

You must decide which evidence is appropriate. There are two main types – objective and subjective evidence.

Objective evidence

This means evidence which confirms you have undertaken the activity. So, in the case of CPD evidence, for example, you may use a programme from a study day you have attended. It is the preferred method of evidence for a portfolio.

Subjective evidence

This is usually self-reporting of having completed an activity or task. For some activities this will be the only way of providing that evidence – for example, if you have received feedback from others. This is often given informally and verbally, therefore the only log of this feedback may be your record of this.

Throughout your career you may undertake a number of types of learning, both work-based and formal. Each of the activities in Table 10.2 presents itself with an opportunity to provide evidence for revalidation.

Recording conversations

You will have conversations as part of your day-to-day work, so it is worthwhile considering how these can be logged as evidence within your portfolio. Consider if you can use what has been said to meet the revalidation requirements. You may be able to use this as evidence of feedback, or it may be something you then reflect on.

The best way to do this is:

● Jot it down at the time or as close to the time as possible – and consider the use of a diary or journal (see section below).

Table 10.2 Activities and examples of portfolio evidence

Activity	Examples of portfolio evidence
New role or responsibilities	Objective: a copy of your job description or feedback from others on your practice. Subjective: any reflection on how you have developed as a result of your new role and responsibilities as well as recognizing any changes made to your practice.
Managing a project	Objective: this could include any project plans, Gantt charts or action plans. You can also include evidence by asking for written feedback from a number of sources – e.g. project team, manager, staff etc. Subjective: you can log your learning as CPD, reflect on the effectiveness of the project and identify any future learning.
Patient-centred care	Objective: you can keep blank copies of any patient information, care plans or documentation you have developed. Subjective: you can use feedback from patients or service users as long as this is anonymized (see Chapter 5). You can also use any reflections on care you have delivered.

● Use quotation marks, where applicable, to strengthen the feed-back – for example, you could note down a quote of your manager giving you feedback that you were 'very clear and concise' in the way you spoke to those relatives.

Case study 1

You receive some comments from another member of staff that you were an 'excellent role model' when dealing with some conflict within your area.

You could consider using this comment to reflect on:
Why you dealt with this conflict in the way you did?
What attributes you demonstrated that made you be viewed as a role model?
How you can improve this in the future?

You can then use this conversation as evidence of your CPD, practice-related feedback and/or to write one of your reflections to meet revalidation requirements.

It is also important to keep a log of your reflective discussion and confirmation, and you must use the NMC templates for both of these. However, you may want to consider recording any additional key points plus any actions you want to take as a result of these meetings. This information should link to your ongoing professional development and appraisal.

Journaling

This means keeping a log of any evidence on a daily basis. A log can be a good way of starting your portfolio. It is simply a written record of your thoughts, experiences and observations which is recorded contemporaneously. This is an informal way of recording your learning, CPD, feedback and reflections without worrying too much about how this is worded. You can collect these on a regular basis then use this information as evidence for your portfolio. You can link to this evidence or transfer some of this evidence onto the most up-to-date NMC forms and templates. A journal can be a diary or paper journal, it can also be an electronic record kept on your mobile device or computer; however you have to remember the principles of data protection as outlined below.

Confidentiality and data protection

As a registrant you have a professional duty of confidentiality, as you are bound by the Code (NMC 2015a) and, in particular, Section 9, which states you must respect people's right to privacy and confidentiality. You have a common law duty of confidentiality where you are not allowed to disclose personal information to anyone outside the team providing care unless they have the express consent of the person, or there is an overriding public interest (Scottish Executive 2003). However, for the purposes of revalidation evidence you should never disclose personal or identifiable information under any circumstances within your portfolio.

The Information Commissioner's Office (ICO) has specific responsibilities for the promotion and enforcement of the Data Protection Act. The ICO has published guidance on data protection and anonymization, which is available on their website. Personal data has to be processed in line with the eight principles of data protection

Table 10.3 Principles of data protection

The eight principles of data protection are that information is:

1. Used fairly and lawfully.
2. Used for limited, specifically stated purposes.
3. Used in a way that is adequate, relevant and not excessive.
4. Accurate.
5. Kept for no longer than is absolutely necessary.
6. Handled according to people's data protection rights.
7. Kept safe and secure.
8. Not transferred outside the European Economic Area without adequate protection.

(ICO 2015)

(see Table 10.3). Some of the information you are expected to collect and record as part of reflective discussion and confirmation is classed as personal data.

Examples of personal data may include the reflective discussion partner or confirmer's:

● Name
● Address
● Full postcode
● NMC PIN or other regulatory body registration number (if applicable).

It is up to organizations to consider their own obligations under the Data Protection Act (1998), and they should consider seeking advice that is specific to them from the Information Commissioner's Office in relation to this.

All personal information is held under strict legal and ethical obligations of confidentiality. Information given in confidence should not be used or disclosed in a form that might identify someone without their consent (Scottish Executive 2003). It is important when recording CPD, feedback, reflective accounts, or when having a reflective and confirmation discussion that you are aware of anything that may be used to identify a patient or colleague, directly or indirectly. For example – rare diseases, drug treatments or specific details which may only apply to a small number of the population which may allow individuals to be identified.

Anonymization

Data is said to be anonymized when items such as name, address, full postcode and any other detail that might identify a person are removed; the data about a person cannot be identified by the recipient of the information; and the theoretical probability of the person's identity being discovered is extremely small. For the purposes of your portfolio and for revalidation you must anonymize any information fully before including it. Any data which may be contained on the reflective and the confirmation discussion form which is not anonymized must be stored securely.

Case study 2

Myrna Shaw works as a prison nurse. She has collated all of her evidence for revalidation using an electronic portfolio and wonders how she can share this information with her reflective discussion partner and confirmer. Her line manager isn't a registrant, so she will be having her reflective discussion and confirmation meetings with separate people at different times. Myrna also knows her confirmation meeting will be held over video conference (VC) because her line manager works in a different prison, so she also wonders how she will get the necessary forms signed.

When considering this case study you may have considered the following:

Myrna could download and print her reflective accounts for her reflective discussion partner because she is meeting them face-to-face. She could also email the relevant parts of her portfolio to her confirmer for discussion over VC.

The reflective discussion is being held face-to-face, so it is likely that the relevant form can be signed at this meeting. She can then choose to scan this into her portfolio or store this paper document securely instead, ensuring she complies with the eight principles of data protection at all times. Myrna could ask her confirmer to sign this form electronically and could then store this within her electronic portfolio, again ensuring she treats this information as personal data.

If Myrna was in any doubt she could contact her local information governance department or read the most up-to-date guidance on the NMC website for more information (NMC2015e).

Forms and templates

Various NMC forms have been produced and can be downloaded free of charge from the NMC website. At the moment, some of these are mandatory and some are recommended. The NMC do not want these forms currently adapted from the format in which they have provided them. This is because the NMC will continue to update the guidance and make revisions to the forms and templates as necessary, so it is important that nurses and midwives access the most up-to-date versions through the NMC website directly when they are due to revalidate.

NMC verification

The NMC expect any evidence within your portfolio to be kept in English. You can use the checklist available below to confirm you have all of the evidence required to revalidate. The NMC recommend that you keep your revalidation evidence in your portfolio until after your next revalidation. For example, if you revalidate in 2016, they suggest that you should keep your portfolio until after you have revalidated again in 2019 (NMC 2015e). The NMC will select a number of portfolios to verify. If you are selected for verification you will be contacted via email and asked for additional information. At this time you will not be required to upload your entire portfolio, but you will be asked for information about your revalidation evidence. (See the NMC website for more guidance on the verification process.)

Revalidation portfolio checklist

- ✓ Evidence of the required number of practice hours.
- ✓ Evidence of the required amount of CPD (including participatory learning).
- ✓ Evidence of the required number of pieces of practice-related feedback.
- ✓ Copy of your signed and completed reflective discussion form.
- ✓ Copy of your signed and completed confirmation form.
- ✓ Evidence of professional indemnity cover if required. (For revalidation purposes you only need to make a self-declaration that you have appropriate cover. However, if you work outside the NHS you need to check you have appropriate indemnity.)

Celebrating achievements

Remember to reflect regularly on your portfolio by reviewing your progress as this can help you set new goals and reflect and celebrate your achievements. Finding out what you can do already by using the self-assessment referred to in Chapter 4 is a good starting point. In each year of your revalidation cycle, perhaps in line with your annual appraisal, it is worth reviewing all of your evidence to see if it meets the requirements. Make a list of anything you are missing and make a plan as to how you are going to achieve this.

Summary

Creating a portfolio is a good opportunity to review, revisit and develop your practice. This can be used for several purposes, including revalidation. There are many benefits to keeping all of your evidence in one place, providing you consider the appropriate way to store all of this. Either a paper or electronic portfolio can be used for revalidation purposes, and this simply depends on your personal preferences.

Key points

- NMC registrants are advised to maintain a portfolio as evidence for revalidation. If you do not already do this you should start this as soon as possible. This means you have all your evidence together in one place.
- Your evidence should link closely with the themes in the Code (NMC 2015a), and it is advisable to ensure that the four sections are included.
- Consider collecting your revalidation evidence as part of life-long learning recorded within your career-long portfolio.

References

Arnold, E.C. and Boggs, K,U. (2016) *Interpersonal Relationships: Professional Communication Skills for Nurses*, 7th cdn. Missouri: Elsevier.

Atkins, S. and Murphy, K. (1993) Reflection: A review of the literature, *Journal of Advanced Nursing*, 18(8): 1188–92.

Atkins, S. and Shutz, S. (2013) Developing the skills for reflective practice, in C. Bulman and S. Shutz (eds) *Reflective Practice in Nursing*, 4th edn. Oxford: Wiley Blackwell.

Balzer-Riley, J. (2011) *Communication in Nursing*, 7th edn. St Louis, MO: Mosby.

Barnlund, D.C. (2008) A transactional model of communication, in C.D. Mortensen (eds) *Communication theory*, 2nd edn. New Brunswick, NJ: Transaction.

Bateson, G. (1979) *Mind and Nature: A Necessary Unity*. New York: E.P. Dutton.

Biggs, J. (2003) *Teaching for Quality Learning at University*, 2nd edn. Buckingham: SRHE and Open University Press.

Birdwhistell, R.L. (1955) Background to kinesics, *Et cetera*, 13(1): 10–28.

Borrill, C., West, M., Dawson, J. et al. (2002) *Team Working and Effectiveness in Health Care*. Aston: Aston Centre for Health Service Organisation Research, University of Aston.

Boud, D., Keogh, R. and Walker, D. (1985) *Reflection: Turning Experience into Learning*. London: Kogan Page.

Bowman, M. and Addyman, B. (2014) Academic reflective writing: A study to examine its usefulness, *British Journal of Nursing*, 23(6): 304–9.

Brookfield, S.D. (1986) *Understanding and Facilitating Adult Learning: A Comprehensive Analysis of Principles and Effective Practices*. California: Jossey-Bass, Inc.

Bulman, C. and Schutz, S. (eds) (2008) *Reflective Practice in Nursing*, 4th edn. Oxford: Blackwell.

Bulman, C., Lathlean, J. and Gobbi, M. (2012) The concept of reflection in nursing: Qualitative findings on student and teacher perspectives, *Nurse Education Today*, 32(5): e8–e13.

Burgoon, J.K., Guerrero, L.K. and Floyd, K. (2016) *Nonverbal Communication*. New York: Routledge.

Buring, S.M., Bhushan, A., Broeseker, A. et al. (2009) Interprofessional education: Definitions, student competencies, and guidelines for implementation, *American Journal of Pharmaceutical Education*, 73(4): 59.

Burns, S. and Bulman, C. (2000) *Reflective Practice in Nursing*. Oxford: Blackwell Science.

Centre for Advancement of Interprofessional Education (CAIPE) (2002). Available at: http://www.caipe.org.uk (accessed 15 January 2016).

Chapman, A. (2010) *Coaching*. Available at: http://www.businessballs. com/coaching.htm (accessed 12 May 2016).

Clark, A.C. (2010a) How to compile a professional portfolio of practice 2: Structure and building evidence, *Nursing Times*, 106(42): 14–17.

Clark, A.C. (2010b) How to compile a professional portfolio of practice 1: Aims and learning outcomes, *Nursing Times*, 106(41): 12–14.

Clayton, M. (2012) *Brilliant Project Leader: What the Best Project Leaders Know, Do and Say to Get Results, Every Time*. Harlow: Pearson Education Limited.

Coleman, A. (2008) *A Dictionary of Psychology*, 3rd edn. Oxford: Oxford University Press.

Covey, R.S. (2004) *The 7 Habits of Highly Effective People*. London: Simon and Schuster.

Crown (2004) The Shipman Inquiry Chairman: Dame Janet Smith DBE, *Fifth Report – Safeguarding Patients: Lessons from the Past – Proposals for the Future*. Norwich: HMSO.

Cutlip, S.M., Center, A.H. and Broom, G.M. (2006) *Effective Public Relations*, 9th edn. New Jersey: Pearson Prentice Hall.

Daniels, A.C. (2009) *Oops! 13 Management Practices that Waste Time and Money (and What to do Instead)*. Atlanta, GA: Performance Management Publications.

Data Protection Act (1998). Available at: http://www.legislation.gov.uk/ukpga/1998/29/contents (accessed 6 December 2016).

Devenny, B. and Duffy, K. (2013) Person-centred reflective practice, *Nursing Standard*, 28(28): 37–43.

Dewey, J. (1933) *How We Think*. Boston: D.C. Heath and Company.

Doran, G.T. (1981) There's a S.M.A.R.T. way to write management goals and objectives, *Management Review*, 70(11): 35–36.

Driscoll, J. (2007) *Practising Clinical Supervision: A Reflective Approach for Healthcare Professionals*, 2nd edn. Edinburgh: Bailliere Tindall Elsevier.

Entwistle, N. (1981) *Styles of Learning and Teaching: An Integrated Outline of Educational Psychology for Students, Teachers and Lecturers*. Chichester: John Wiley.

Fielden, S.L., Davidson, M.J. and Sutherland, V.J. (2009) Innovations in coaching and mentoring: implications of nurse leadership development, *Health Services Management Research*, 22(2): 92–9.

Fleming, N. and Baume, D. (2006) Learning styles again: VARKing up the right tree!, *Educational Developments*, SEDA Ltd, 7(4): 4–7. Available at: http://www.vark-learn.com/wp-content/uploads/2014/08/Educational-Developments.pdf (accessed 10 January 2016).

Forde, C., McMahon, M. and Reeves, J. (2009) *Putting Together Professional Portfolios*. London: Sage Publishing.

Fowler, J. (2014) Reflection: from staff nurse to nurse consultant. Part 2: What is reflection?, *British Journal of Nursing*, 23(4): 232.

General Medical Council (GMC) and Nursing and Midwifery Council (NMC) (2015) *Openness and Honesty When Things go Wrong: The Professional Duty of Candour*. London: General Medical Council and Nursing and Midwifery Council.

Available at: http://www.gmc-uk.org/DoC_guidance_englsih. pdf_61618688.pdf (accessed 14 February 2016).

Gibbs, G. (1988) *Learning by Doing: A Guide to Teaching and Learning Methods*. Oxford: Oxford Polytechnic Further Education Unit.

Gibson, C., Hardy III, J.H. and Buckly, M.R. (2014) Understanding the role of networking in organizations, *Career Development International*, 19(2): 146–61.

Glazzard, J., Denby, N. and Price, J. (2014) *Learning to Teach*. Maidenhead: Open University Press.

Goleman, D. (1996) *Emotional Intelligence: Why it can Matter More than IQ*. London: Bloomsbury Publishing plc.

Grainger, A. (2010) What if . . . ? Reflective practice, *British Journal of Healthcare Assistants*, 4(5): 226–8.

Helen and Douglas House (2015) *Clinical Supervision Toolkit*. Oxford: Helen and Douglas House.

Honey, P. and Mumford, A. (1986a) *The Manual of Learning Styles*. Maidenhead: Peter Honey Associates.

Honey, P. and Mumford, A. (1986b) *Learning Styles Questionnaire*. Maidenhead: Peter Honey Associates.

Hurley, J. (2008) The necessity, barriers and ways forward to meet user-based needs for emotionally intelligent nurses, *Journal of Psychiatric Mental Health Nursing*, 15(5): 379–85.

Information Commissioners Office (ICO) (2015) *Data Protection*. Available at: https://www.gov.uk/data-protection/the-data-protection-act (accessed 21 May 2016).

Jasper, M. (2006) *Professional Development, Reflection and Decision-making*. Oxford: Blackwell Publishing.

Jasper, M. (2013) *Beginning Reflective Practice*, 2nd edn. Cheltenham: Nelson Thornes.

Johns, C. (2000) *Becoming a Reflective Practitioner*. Oxford: Blackwell Science.

Juwah, C., MacFarlane-Dick, D., Matthew, B. et al. (2004) *Enhancing Student Learning through Effective Formative Feedback*.

York: Higher Education Academy. Available at: https://www.
heacademy.ac.uk/sites/default/files/resources/id353_senlef_guide.
pdf (accessed 26 May 2016).

Knowles M.S., Holton, E.F. and Swanson, R.A. (2005) *The Adult
Learner: The Definitive Classic in Adult Education and Human
Resource Development*, 6th edn. Amsterdam: Elsevier.

Kolb, D.A. (1984) *Experiential Learning: Experience as the Source
of Learning and Development*. New Jersey: Prentice-Hall.

Kolyva, K. (2015) How reflection can raise standards of nursing
care, *Nursing Times*, 111(44): 16.

Madden, C.A. and Mitchell, V.A. (1993) *Professions, Standards
and Competence: A Survey of Continuing Education for the
Professions*. University of Bristol: Department for Continuing
Education.

Masella, R.S. (2007) Renewing professionalism in dental education:
Overcoming the market environment, *Journal of Dental Education*, 71(2): 205–16.

McCabe, C. and Timmins, F. (2013) *Communication Skills for Nursing
Practice*, 2nd edn. London: Palgrave Macmillan.

McGill, I. and Brockbank, A. (2004) *The Action Learning Handbook:
Powerful Techniques for Education, Professional Development
and Training*. London: Routledge.

McKeachie, W.J. (2002) *McKeachie's Teaching Tips: Strategies,
Research, and Theory for College and University Teachers*, 11th
edn. Massachusetts: Houghton Mifflin Company.

Mehrabian, A. and Ferris, S.R. (1967) Inference of attitudes from non-
verbal communication in two channels, *Journal of Consulting
Psychology*, 31(3): 48–258.

Merriam, S.B. and Caffarella, R.S. (1999) *Learning in Adulthood:
A Comprehensive Guide*, 2nd edn. California: John Wiley and
Sons, Inc.

Middleton, H. (2011) How to build your professional portfolio (and
why you should), *Clinical Pharmacist*, 1 Jan. Available at: http://
www.pharmaceutical-journal.com/careers/career-feature/

how-to-build-your-professional-portfolio-and-why-you-should/
11072302.article (accessed 20 May 2016).

Miller, G.R. and Nicholson, H.E. (1976) *Communication Inquiry: A Perspective on a Process*. Reading: Addison Wesley.

Mills, J.E., Francis, K.L. and Bonner, A. (2005) Mentoring, clinical supervision and preceptoring: clarifying the conceptual definitions for Australian rural nurses. A review of the literature, *Rural and Remote Health* (Online), 5(3): 410. Available at: http://www.rrh.org.au/articles/subviewnew.asp?ArticleID=410 (accessed 23 January 2016).

MindTools.com (2016) SWOT Analysis [online]. Available at: https://www.mindtools.com/pages/article/newTMC_05.htm (accessed 13 July 2016).

Nath, V., Seale, B. and Kaur, M. (2014) *Medical Revalidation from Compliance to Commitment*. London: The King's Fund.

Nicol, J.S. and Dosser, I. (2016) Understanding reflective practice, *Nursing Standard*, 30(36): 34–40.

Nursing and Midwifery Council (NMC) (2006) *Preceptorship Guidance*, NMC Circular 21/2006 SAT/gl October 3. London: NMC.

Nursing and Midwifery Council (NMC) (2008a) *Standards for Medicine Administration*. London: NMC.

Nursing and Midwifery Council (NMC) (2008b) *PREP Standards*. London: NMC.

Nursing and Midwifery Council (NMC) (2008c) *Standards to Support Learning and Assessment in Practice*. London: NMC.

Nursing and Midwifery Council (NMC) (2011) *The PREP Handbook*. London: NMC.

Nursing and Midwifery Council (NMC) (2015a) *The Code: Professional Standards of Practice and Behaviour for Nurses and Midwives*. London: NMC.

Nursing and Midwifery Council (NMC) (2015b) *Annual Fitness to Practise Report 2014–2015*. London: NMC. Available at: https://www.nmc.org.uk/globalassets/sitedocuments/annual_reports_and_accounts/ftpannualreports/annual-ftp-report-2014-2015.pdf (accessed 15 December 2015).

Nursing and Midwifery Council (NMC) (2015c) *Raising Concerns: Guidance for Nurses and Midwives.* London: NMC.

Nursing and Midwifery Council (NMC) (2015d) *Social Networking Guidance.* London: NMC.

Nursing and Midwifery Council (NMC) (2015e) *How to Revalidate with the NMC.* London: NMC.

Nursing and Midwifery Council (NMC) (2015f) *Information for Confirmers.* London: NMC.

Nursing and Midwifery Council (NMC) (2015g) *Employers' Guide to Revalidation.* London: NMC.

Nursing and Midwifery Council (NMC) (2016a) *Registering as a Nurse or Midwife in the UK for Applicants Trained in the EU or EEA.* Available at: http://www.nmc.org.uk/globalassets/sitedocuments/ registration/registering-as-a-nurse-or-midwife-in-the-uk-for- applicants-trained-in-eea-jan2016.pdf (accessed 20 January 2016).

Nursing and Midwifery Council (NMC) (2016b) *Supervisor of Mid- wives: How They can Help You.* Available at: http://www.nmc. org.uk/globalassets/sitedocuments/midwifery-reports/nmc- supervisor-of-midwives-how-they-can-help-you.pdf (accessed 22 January 2016).

Nursing and Midwifery Order (2001). Available at: https://www.nmc. org.uk/about-us/our-legal-framework/our-order-and-rules/ (accessed 10 July 2016).

Oelofsen, N. (2012) Developing practical reflective skills (1/2): personal learning, *British Journal of Healthcare Assistants,* 6(6): 294–7.

Patrick, F. (2011) *Handbook of Research on Improving Learning and Motivation.* Hershey, PA: IGI Global.

Patterson, M.L. and Edinger, J.A. (2014) A functional analysis of space in social interaction, in A.W. Siegman and S. Feldstein (eds) *Nonverbal Behavior and Communication,* 2nd edn. New York: Psychology Press.

Pendleton, D., Scofield, T., Tate, P. et al. (1984) *The Consultation: An Approach to Learning and Teaching.* Oxford: Oxford University Press.

Petrie, P. (1997) *Communicating with Children and Adults: Interpersonal Skills for Early Years and Play Work.* London: Arnold.

Pitts, J. (2010) Portfolios, personal development and reflective practice, in T. Swanwick (ed.) *Understanding Medical Education: Evidence, Theory and Practice.* Oxford: Wiley-Blackwell.

Quinn, F. (1998) Reflection and reflective practice, in F. Quinn (ed.) *Continuing Professional Development in Nursing: A Guide for Practitioners and Educators.* Cheltenham: Stanley Thornes Ltd.

Race, P. (2001) *2000 Tips for Trainers and Staff Developers.* London: Routledge.

Ramsden, P. (ed.) (1988) *Improving Learning: New Perspectives.* London: Kogan Page.

Rosdahl, C.B. and Kowalski, M.T. (2008) *Textbook of Basic Nursing,* 9th edn. Philadelphia: Lippincott Williams and Wilkins.

Royal College of Nursing (RCN) (2009) *The Knowledge and Skills Framework and Appraisal Guidance for Members and Employers Outside of the NHS.* London: RCN.

Scholes, J., Webb, C., Gray, M. et al. (2004) Making portfolios work in practice, *Journal of Advanced Nursing,* 46(6): 595–603.

Schön, D. (1983) *The Reflective Practitioner.* New York: Basic Books.

Scottish Executive (2003) *NHS Code of Practice on Protecting Patient Confidentiality.* Edinburgh: NHS Scotland. Available at: http://www.ed.ac.uk/files/imports/fileManager/NHS%20Code%20of%20Practice%20on%20Protecting%20Patient%20Confidentiality.pdf (accessed 3 December 2015).

Scottish Executive (2005) *Networking and Learning for Practice Management, Appraisal for Practice Managers in Scotland.* Edinburgh: Scottish Executive. Available at: www.scotland.gov.uk/Publications/2005/06/09104542/45445 (accessed 11 February 2016).

The Scottish Government (2008) *Supporting the Development of Advanced Nursing Practice: A Toolkit Approach.* Edinburgh: The Scottish Government. Available at: http://www.advancedpractice.

scot.nhs.uk/media/1371/supporting%20the%20development%20 of%20advanced%20nursing%20practice.pdf (accessed 20 December 2015).

The Scottish Government (2012) *Professionalism in Nursing, Midwifery and the Allied Health Professions in Scotland: A Report to the Coordinating Council for the NMAHP Contribution to the Healthcare Quality Strategy for NHSScotland.* Edinburgh: The Scottish Government. Available at: http://www.gov.scot/ resource/0039/00396525.pdf (accessed 12 January 2016).

Siegel, D.J. (2007) *The Mindful Brain: Reflection and Attunement in the Cultivation of Well-being.* London: W.W. Norton and Company.

Silberman, M.L. and Auerbach, C. (1998) *Active Training: A Handbook of Techniques, Designs, Case Examples, and Tips*, 2nd edn. California: John Wiley and Sons, Inc.

Skills for Care (2007) *Providing Effective Supervision: A Workforce Development Tool, including a Unit of Competence and Supporting Guidance.* Leeds: Skills for Care. Available at: http:// www.skillsforcare.org.uk/Document-library/Finding-and-keeping-workers/Supervision/Providing-Effective-Supervision. pdf (accessed 30 January 2016).

Smith, A. and Desai, S. (2010) Prescribing practice from the employer's perspective: The rationale for CPD within non-medical prescribing, in M. Waite and J. Keenan (eds) *CPD for Non-medical Prescribers: A Practical Guide.* Oxford: Blackwell Publishing.

Stone, D. and Heen, S. (2015) *Thanks for the Feedback: The Science and Art of Receiving Feedback.* New York: Penguin Group.

Stonehouse, D. (2011) Using reflective practice to ensure high standards of care, *British Journal of Healthcare Assistants*, 5(6): 299–302.

Thatch, E.C. (2002) The impact of executive coaching and 360 feedback on leadership effectiveness, *Leadership and Organization Development Journal*, 23(4): 205–14.

Thompson, N. (2009) *People Skills*, 3rd edn. Hampshire: Palgrave Macmillan.

Timmins, F. and Duffy, A. (2011) *Writing your Nursing Portfolio: A Step-by-step Guide.* Maidenhead: Open University Press.

Titchen, A. (2000) *Professional Craft Knowledge in Patient-centred Nursing.* Kidlington: Ashdale Press.

Tsang, A.K.L. (2010) The evolving professional (EP) concept as a framework for the scholarship of teaching and learning, *International Journal for the Scholarship of Teaching and Learning,* 4(1): Article 12. Available at: http://www.georgiasouthern.edu/ ijsotl (accessed 26 May 2016).

UK Government (2007) *Trust, Assurance and Safety – The Regulation of Health Professionals in the 21st Century.* London: Stationery Office. Available at: https://www.gov.uk/government/ publications/trust-assurance-and-safety-the-regulation-of-health-professionals-in-the-21st-century (accessed 22 December 2015).

Walsh, K. (2005) The rules, *British Medical Journal,* 331(7516): 574.

Westwick, J. (2013) Understanding proxemics through restrooms: a 'hands-off' approach to personal space and communication, *Communication and Theater Association of Minnesota Journal,* 40: 59–62. Available at: http://cornerstone.lib.mnsu.edu/cgi/ viewcontent.cgi?article=1077&context=ctamj (accessed 22 May 2016).

Index

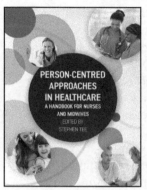

Person-centred approaches in healthcare
A handbook for nurses and midwives

Stephen Tee (Ed)

ISBN: 9780335263585 (Paperback)
eISBN: 9780335263592

2016

Written by practitioners, academics and, more importantly, the people who use health services, this unique text examines the application of person-centred principles across a range of healthcare contexts. It will provide you with the essential skills, techniques and strategies needed to deliver person-centred care.

Patients and service users should be at the heart of healthcare delivery and this book will equip nurses and midwives by connecting the reader to the lived experience of those receiving healthcare. It examines issues across the lifespan and reveals how person-centred care can best be achieved by working in partnership.

After introducing key principles and service design in chapters I and 2, each chapter that follows tackles a different age or disease specific area of care, including:

- Maternity care
- Family care including health visiting
- Adolescent care
- Adult critical care
- Diseases including diabetes and arthritis
- Care for people with long term mental health problems
- Intellectual disabilities
- Care of carers

www.mheducation.co.uk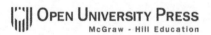

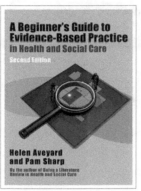

**A BEGINNER'S GUIDE TO EVIDENCE-BASED
PRACTICE IN HEALTH AND SOCIAL CARE**

Second Edition

Helen Aveyard and Pam Sharp

ISBN: 9780335246724 (Paperback)
eBook:

2013

**Have you heard of 'evidence based practice' but don't know what it
means?**
Are you having trouble relating evidence to your practice?

This is **the** book for anyone who has ever wondered what evidence based
practice is or how to relate it to practice. Fully updated in this brand new
edition, this book is simple and easy to understand – and designed to help
those new to the topic to apply the concept to their practice and learning
with ease.

Key features:

- Additional material on literature reviews and searching for literature
- Even more examples for health and social care practice
- Extra material on qualitative research and evidence based practice
- Expanded section on hierarchies of evidence and how to use them

www.mheducation.co.uk

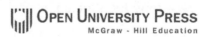

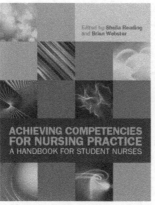

**ACHIEVING COMPETENCIES FOR
NURSING PRACTICE**
A Handbook for Student Nurses

Sheila Reading and Brian James Webster
(Eds)

9780335246748 (Paperback)
2014

eBook also available

Achieving the NMC Competencies is an ongoing requirement that nurses
work towards across all three years of pre-registration study. This book
illuminates what students need to understand about each of the
competencies and illustrates how best to achieve them in training and
practice.

Key features:

- Each chapter tackles a different competency
- Uses activities and examples to help readers get to grips with the
  competency and relevant NMC requirements
- The book is very interactive and offers lot of portfolio activities for
  students to try, and use to demonstrate competency as they build a
  portfolio evidence

www.mheducation.co.uk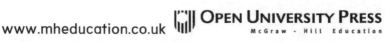